$12.95

The
HIGH BLOOD PRESSURE
Book

A SERIES OF BOOKS ABOUT MEDICAL CARE

ROBERT J. GLASER, M.D., *Editor*

The High Blood Pressure Book by Edward D. Freis, M.D., and Gina Bari Kolata

The Arthritis Book by Ephraim P. Engleman, M.D., and Milton Silverman, Ph.D.

Your Coronary Arteries by J. Willis Hurst, M.D., and Dorothy S. Luciano, Ph.D.

Other titles to be announced

The HIGH BLOOD PRESSURE Book

A Guide for Patients and Their Families

by
EDWARD D. FREIS, M.D.,
and
GINA BARI KOLATA

with a foreword by
ROBERT J. GLASER, M.D.

PAINTER HOPKINS PUBLISHERS
Sausalito California

Illustrated by Richard Roesener, San Francisco, California.

Printed in the United States of America. Published simultaneously in Canada by Clarke, Irwin & Company, Limited, Toronto and Vancouver.

For information contact Painter Hopkins Publishers, P.O. Box 1829, Sausalito, California 94965.

Library of Congress Cataloging in Publication Data

Freis, Edward D

The high blood pressure book.
1. Hypertension. I. Kolata, Gina Bari, joint author.
II. Title. [DNLM: 1. Hypertension—Popular works.
WG340.3 F866h]
RC685.H8F65 616.1'32 79-10442

ISBN 0-525-12472-1

1 2 3 4 5 6 7 8 9 10

To Willa Freis and Bill Kolata

Most people with high blood pressure have no symptoms warning them that anything is wrong. But the pressure that the blood exerts on their arteries is dangerously high. Physicians have agreed to call all blood pressures above a certain range "high" to indicate that people who have such blood pressures are at risk of developing heart attacks, strokes, or congestive heart failure. Fortunately, these serious consequences of high blood pressure can often be prevented if the pressure is lowered by medical treatment.

CONTENTS

FOREWORD

This volume on high blood pressure is the first in a series of short books about important common diseases, written by distinguished experts and designed to give patients authentic information about their disease—its origin, course, treatment, and outlook. The book is similarly intended for the families of patients. In the case of any chronic disease, whatever its manifestations, family members are inevitably involved, directly or indirectly; they have the opportunity to provide important support, both emotional and practical. Better understanding on the part of all concerned can only be beneficial.

The information in this book will complement that given the patient by his or her physician. Because of the demanding responsibilities every busy physician confronts, he or she cannot spend long periods explaining the many ramifications of a disease as complex as high blood pressure. On the other hand, once the patient is self-informed as a result of reading this volume, he can direct remaining questions toward the physician in concise form and receive answers in an efficient manner.

High blood pressure, or hypertension, affects millions of men and women around the world. A common disease with a high incidence, it is identified with complications that are serious, often life-threatening, and frequently fatal. Nonetheless, it is only in recent times that we have come to understand the cause of some of the less-common forms of the disease. Effective treatment, well described in this book, is an even more recent addition to the physician's armamentarium, and, fortunately, treatment is successful in the commonest type of high blood pressure, known as essential hypertension, even though its cause remains to be elucidated.

Because hypertension is "silent," or asymptomatic, initially, or even for relatively long periods, it used to be a disease for which physicians did not generally recommend treatment until symptoms appeared. Patients often did not seek medical care either because they were unaware that they had the disease or because, even knowing of its presence, they were free of symptoms.

As a result of the Framingham study (described in Chapter 4) and other investigative efforts following World War II, it has become clear that high blood pressure poses a distinct threat to an individual's well-being and long-term outlook even when asymptomatic. Fortunately, concomitant with heightened appreciation by physicians of the dangers of hypertension, the discovery of drugs effective in lowering the blood pressure has afforded a means of combatting the problem.

Today, in a small percentage of cases, cure is possible. For most of the very large proportion of patients whose disease is not curable in the definitive sense, the drugs now available, used in an appropriate manner, usually make reduction of blood pressure achievable, and they alter the outlook dramatically for the better. Further, ongoing widespread laboratory research continues to add to our understanding of the mechanisms by which high blood pressure produces its deleterious effects and unveils other agents even more effective in treatment than those already available.

It is now clear that the early diagnosis of hypertension is critical, because treatment initiated at the onset of the disease significantly improves the prognosis, or outlook. The older idea that treatment was not indicated in the absence of overt symptoms was wrong. Yet it is often difficult for patients to understand why they should bother with medication when they feel well. Experience indicates that as many as 50 percent of patients fail to comply with the treatment plans prescribed by their physicians. To at least some extent, this failure to follow instructions that promise to increase longevity as well as the quality of life reflects lack of understanding on the part of the patient.

It is reasonable to assume that if patients with hypertension—and their families who are inevitably involved with them in sickness and in health—understand the nature of hypertension, and the effect of treatment or lack of it on the course of the disease, they will exert every effort to comply with the treatments prescribed by their physicians. This book makes that requisite understanding available in layman's language.

Its senior author, Dr. Edward D. Freis, has contributed in large measure to the progress in our understanding of hypertension, and particularly to the demonstration of the value of treatment in preventing complications and increasing longevity in those afflicted with elevated blood pressure. A graduate of the Columbia University College of Physicians and Surgeons, Dr. Freis received his clinical training in internal medicine at the Massachusetts Memorial Hospital and Boston City Hospital, two major teaching services of the Boston University Medical School. As noted in this book, he participated in some of the pioneering studies of antihypertensive drugs, and, after military service and completion of his clinical training, he moved to Washington, D.C., where he joined the faculty of the Georgetown University School of Medicine. He rose through the academic ranks, and since 1957 has been professor of medicine. He is also chief of both the university's cardiovascular research laboratory and the hypertension clinic, and is a senior medical investigator at the Veterans Administration Hospital.

The recipient of many honors and awards, including the Lasker Award, Dr. Freis is a member of many learned societies. Of particular note in connection with this book is the fact that Dr. Freis directed a landmark study, carried out nationally, that had much to do with confirming the importance of early diagnosis and treatment of hypertension.

Gina Bari Kolata, the co-author, is a highly regarded science writer. A native of Baltimore, she was graduated from the University of Maryland, where she received a B.S. degree in microbiology in 1969, and an M.S. in applied mathematics in 1973. Ms. Kolata has published widely; her contributions have appeared in *The Nation, The Washington Post,* Funk & Wagnall's *Yearbook,* and *La Recherche,* among others. In 1977 she received the Alton Blakeslee Award from the American Heart Association in recognition of a series of nine articles published in *Science* on heart disease. This series also led to an award to Ms. Kolata from the American

Medical Writers Association. For the past six years, she has been a staff member of *Science,* the journal of the American Association for the Advancement of Science.

Robert J. Glaser, M.D.
Consulting Professor of Medicine,
formerly Vice President of
Medical Affairs and
Dean of the School of Medicine,
Stanford University

PREFACE

This is a book about high blood pressure—a disease with devastating effects on the lives of many Americans. Directly and indirectly, high blood pressure kills or disables more Americans than any other medical condition.

But the tide may be turning. In 1971, the U.S. Department of Health, Education, and Welfare established the National High Blood Pressure Education Program. Since then, more and more people are becoming aware of the dangers of high blood pressure and are being treated. Recently, physicians have begun to see evidence that this increased awareness of the importance of controlling high blood pressure may be paying off. The death rates from the two major consequences of high blood pressure—diseases of the heart and strokes—have begun to decline.

Between 1973 and the first nine months of 1977, the number of deaths due to diseases of the heart decreased by 8 percent. In the same period, deaths due to strokes decreased by 16.6 percent. These decreases constitute a saving of about 300,000 lives.

In this book, we will explain the current thinking among medical experts on high blood pressure—what it is, why it is dangerous, how it is treated, and what the side effects of the medications are. We will also discuss such controversial matters as whether cutting out salt, reducing weight, relaxing, or exercising can prevent or cure high blood pressure. We will present information that patients are rarely told, such as the fact that a few patients can eventually reduce their doses of medication (under the supervision of their physicians) and still maintain a lowered blood pressure.

It is our opinion that the well-informed patient is the best patient, the most likely to understand and follow instructions, and the most apt to keep his blood pressure under good control. Therefore, we have tried to be completely honest about what is and what is not known about high blood pressure and have tried always to separate fact from emotion.

If there is one message we wish to convey, it is that *the dire consequences of high blood pressure are largely preventable.* Although we do not know what causes most cases of high blood pressure or whether it is preventable, we do know that high blood pressure can be controlled and that when it is controlled its toll of death and disablement is reduced. We believe that the death rate from diseases of the heart and from strokes will decline still further and we hope that our book will explain how and why the treatment of high blood pressure can enable the hypertensive patient to live a longer and healthier life.

April, 1979

Edward D. Freis, M.D.
Gina Bari Kolata

The HIGH BLOOD PRESSURE Book

CHAPTER 1

WHAT IS HIGH BLOOD PRESSURE?

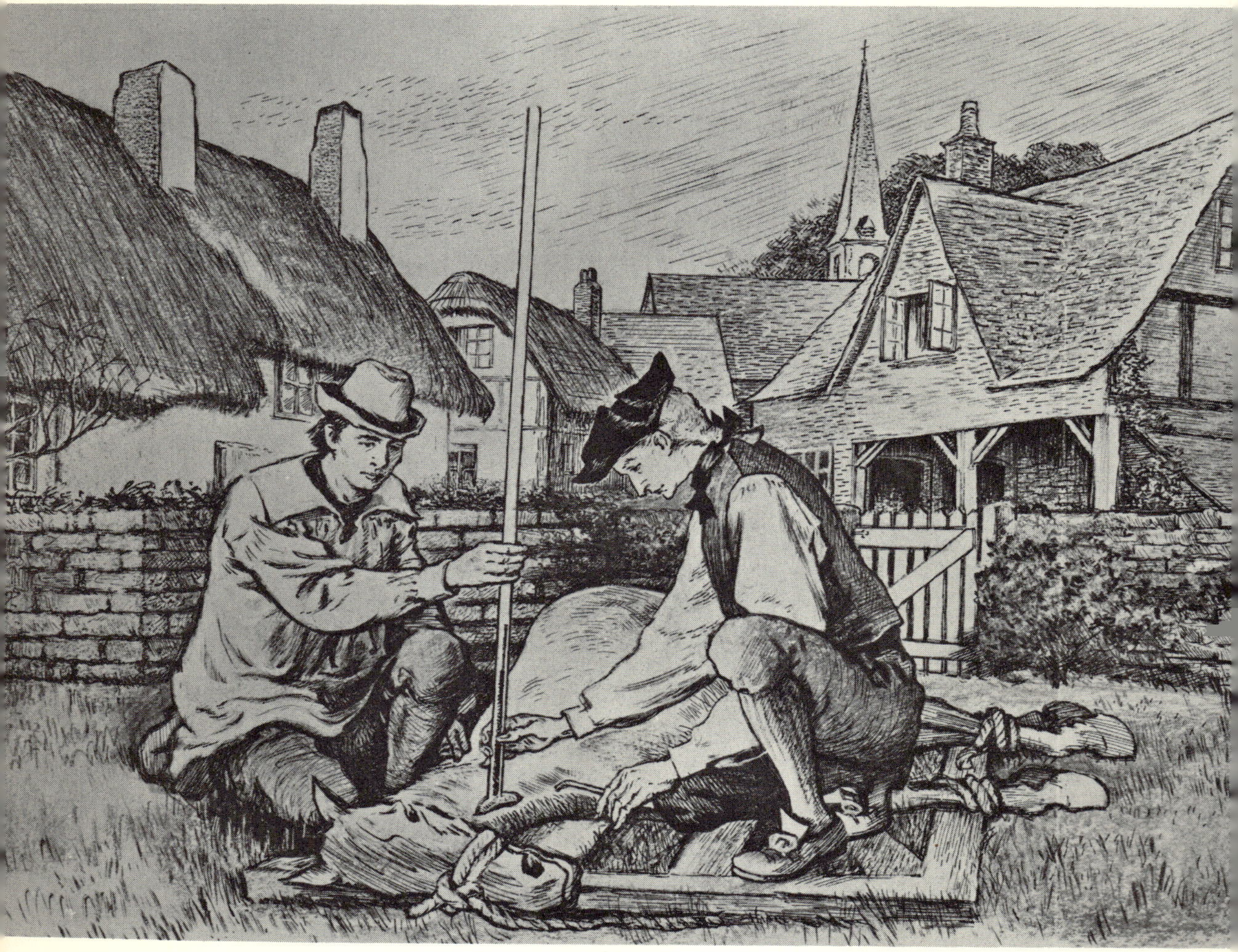

Stephen Hales, "the father of blood pressure," made the first measurement of blood pressure in 1711. He did so in the carotid artery of a horse. Hales was an Anglican minister in Middlesex, England, who liked to experiment in natural science. (the Bettmann Archive.)

High blood pressure is the major cause of death and disablement in the United States. It strikes more Americans than any of the other great crippling and killing diseases. Whereas approximately 3 million, or 1 in 35, Americans have cancer, the National Heart, Lung, and Blood Institute estimates that 35 million, or *1 in every 6,* suffer from definite high blood pressure. High blood pressure is a disease of the young as well as the old, women as well as men, whites as well as blacks, rich as well as poor.

Although all are vulnerable to high blood pressure, the disease takes an even more terrible toll of blacks than whites. Black Americans are 50 percent more likely to have high blood pressure than whites and black women are most likely of all to have the disease. By the time they reach age sixty-five, nearly 50 percent of black men and 60 percent of black women have high blood pressure

And yet for a national health problem of such proportions, high blood pressure plays a remarkably small role in the public consciousness. This is because it is a disease that initially has few or no visible symptoms, and because its effects often appear in its contribution to related and more evident illnesses. It is for most of its course a silent disease.

For this reason, many people who suffer from high blood pressure do not know that they have it. Moreover, many of those whose high blood pressure has been diagnosed do not seek adequate treatment. It is estimated that only one-third of the people who have high blood pressure are being treated, and only half of those being treated follow their physicians' recommendations rigorously enough to bring their blood pressures under control.

Yet uncontrolled high blood pressure is dangerous. An increase in blood pressure increases the risk of dying from

PREVALENCE OF SELECTED CHRONIC DISEASES *(In millions of patients)*

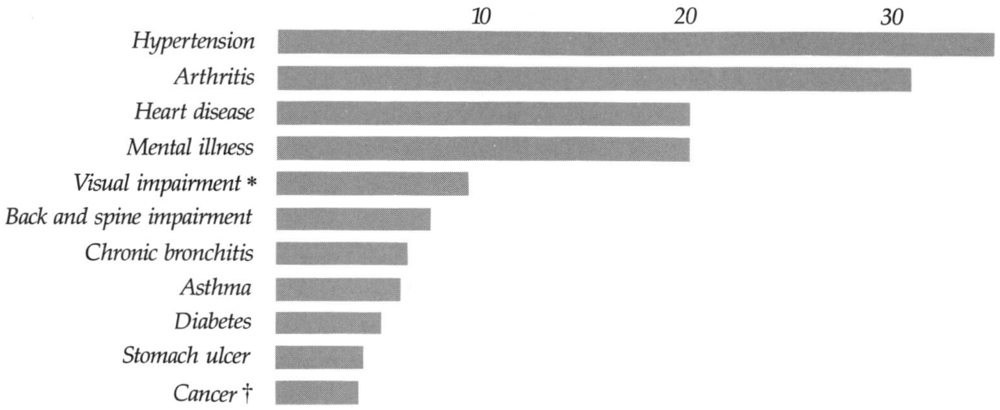

SOURCES: 1978 approximations from the National Center for Health Statistics; National Heart, Lung, and Blood Institute; National Cancer Institute; Arthritis Foundation; American Cancer Society; and National Institute of Arthritis, Metabolism, and Digestive Diseases.

* Impairments not correctable by glasses.

† Nonmelanoma skin cancers not included.

strokes, heart attacks, heart failure, or kidney failure. In a classic twelve-year study undertaken by the Public Health Service in Framingham, Massachusetts, in which a total of 5,209 men and women between the ages of thirty-five and seventy-four were examined, the health records of those with normal blood pressure and those with high blood pressure were compared. *It was found that the high-blood-pressure group had three times as many heart attacks, more than six times as much heart failure, and more than seven times as many strokes as those with normal blood pressure.*

Ironically, death due to high blood pressure is largely preventable. Only rarely is it impossible to bring high blood pressure under some sort of control, and once high blood pressure is controlled the threat of kidney failure, heart failure, strokes, and possibly heart attacks is greatly diminished.

Medical investigators have learned a great deal about the probable causes of high blood pressure and what can be done to control it. We will be sharing these findings with you in subsequent chapters. But in order to help you understand the points we will be making later, we will begin with some basic background information. We will start with a simple description of how the heart and circulatory system work, and then turn to an explanation of how the body controls the blood pressure, how doctors measure blood pressure, and how medical investigators define *high* blood pressure.

Before beginning, we wish to call your attention to a matter of word usage that sometimes causes confusion. Physicians usually refer to high blood pressure as *hypertension.* This word refers only to the tension (pressure) in the blood vessels; it has nothing to do with psychological stress or tension. In this book we will follow standard medical practice and use the terms "hypertension" and "high blood pressure" interchangeably.

The Heart and the Circulatory System

No man-made pump can rival the heart in endurance and efficiency. Although only the size of a person's fist, the heart pumps about 40,000 gallons (160,000 liters) of blood each day through vessels that total 60,000 miles (100,000 kilometers) in length. It accomplishes this awesome task by contracting 100,000 times each day. When the heart muscle contracts, it forces the blood out of the heart into the arteries. When the heart muscle relaxes, the chamber is again filled with blood returning from the veins. These alternating cycles of contraction and relaxation occur continuously throughout life.

The heart itself consists of not one but two pumps that are separated by a thin wall. The right side of the heart pumps blood to the lungs. This is blood that has already circulated through the body and is depleted of oxygen. After the oxygen-poor blood is replenished with oxygen in the lungs, it enters the left side of the heart. From there it is pumped to the rest of the body.

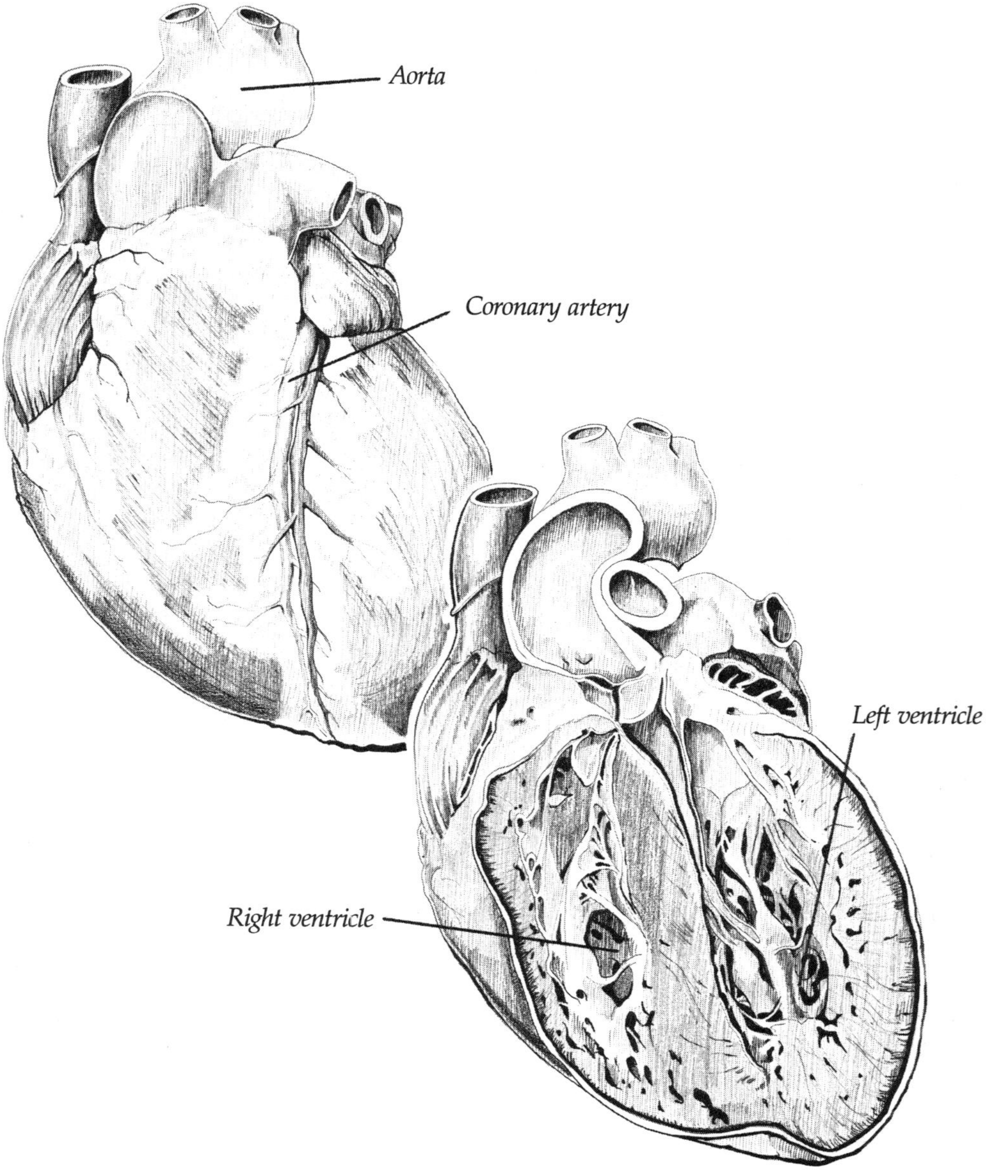

Front view of the heart (left); cross-sectional view (right).

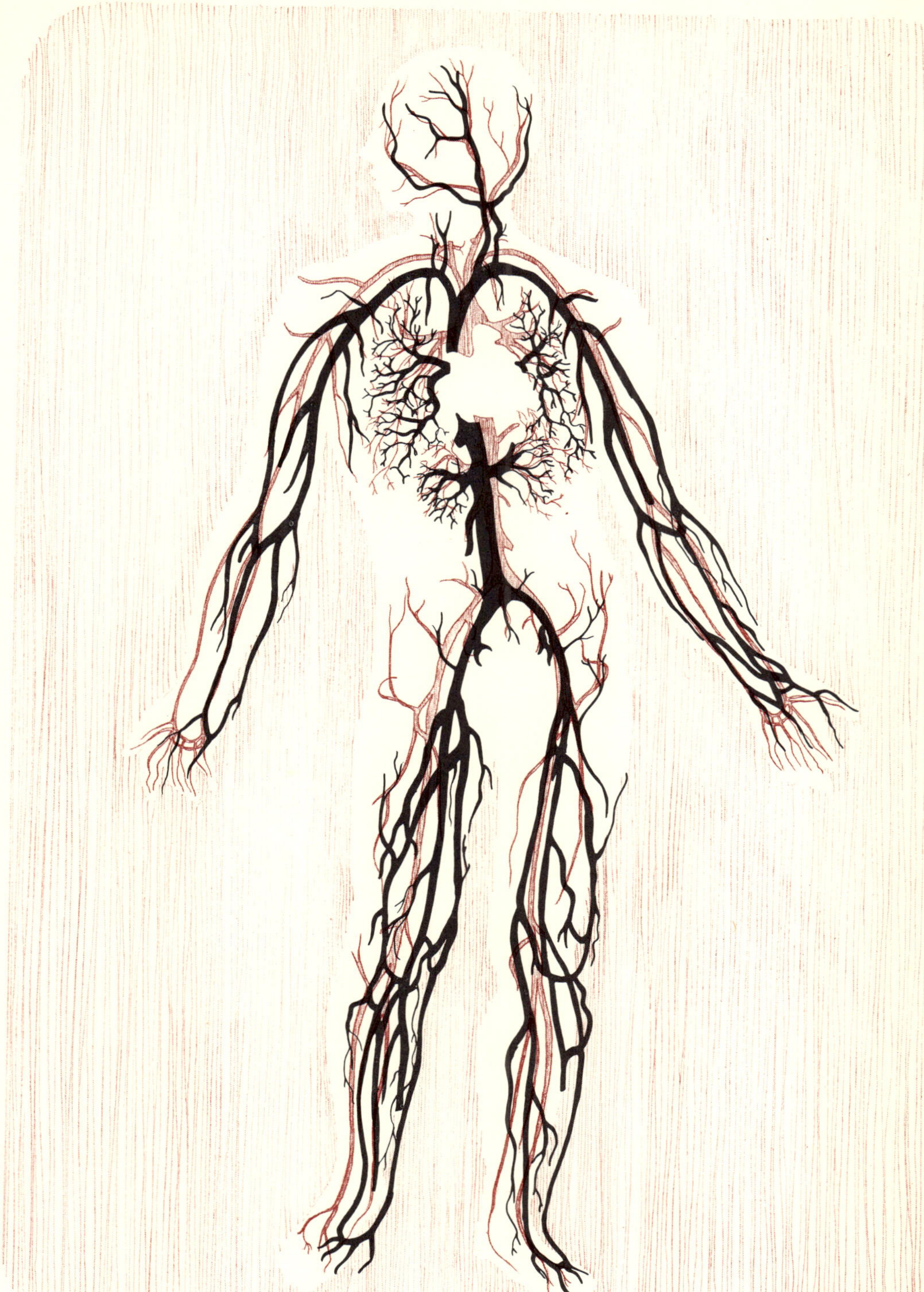

The circulatory system: veins are shown in black; arteries in red.

Oxygen-rich blood leaves the heart through a large artery, called the *aorta*, about the size of a garden hose. This artery then branches into smaller and smaller arteries until they become invisible to the naked eye and have diameters ranging from 10 to 20 ten-thousandths of an inch (0.025–0.05 millimeters). These microscopic vessels are the *arterioles.* As we will explain in a later section, the arterioles play an important role in determining blood pressure.

The arterioles feed blood into still smaller vessels, called *capillaries*, which are so small that blood cells can only go through them single file. Oxygen and nutrients carried by the blood are supplied to the tissues through the capillaries. Then the oxygen-poor blood returns through the veins to the heart, where the whole process starts over.

What Is Blood Pressure?

Blood pressure is the pressure exerted by blood on the walls of the arteries. It is greatest when the heart first contracts, forcing a huge gush of blood into the arteries. The pressure then gradually decreases as the heart relaxes between beats.

You may have noticed that blood pressure is expressed as a ratio of two numbers, such as 120/80. The larger number is a measure of the pressure in the arteries when the heart contracts, a period called *systole* (sis'-toll-ee), and is called *systolic blood pressure.* The smaller number is a measure of the pressure in the arteries when the heart relaxes between beats, a period called *diastole* (die-as'-toll-ee). This pressure is known as *diastolic blood pressure.*

How Is Blood Pressure Measured?

Almost everyone has seen a sphygmomanometer (s'fig'-mo-man-ahmeter)—the instrument generally used to measure blood pressure. It consists of a cloth-covered rubber bladder (called a cuff) that is wrapped around the arm, a bulb used to pump the cuff full of air, and a pressure-measuring device.

Sphygmomanometers measure the blood pressure *indirectly* by relating it to the air pressure in the cuff. A pressure-measuring device is used to measure this air pressure in the cuff. The measuring device is often a tube of mercury. Blood pressure is measured in units of millimeters of mercury, designated mm Hg. A pressure of 120 mm Hg is the pressure needed to push a column of mercury up a tube for a distance of 120 millimeters.

HOW IS BLOOD PRESSURE MEASURED?

When a physician or a technician measures your blood pressure, he wraps the cuff snugly around your arm and pumps air into the cuff until it is so tight that it stops the flow of blood through the arm. While listening through a stethoscope positioned just below the cuff, he drops the pressure in the cuff gradually by releasing air from the cuff. When the pressure in the cuff becomes low enough for blood to begin flowing through your arm just below the cuff, he hears a thumping sound. At this point, the air pressure in the cuff equals the *maximum,* or systolic, blood pressure in the artery.

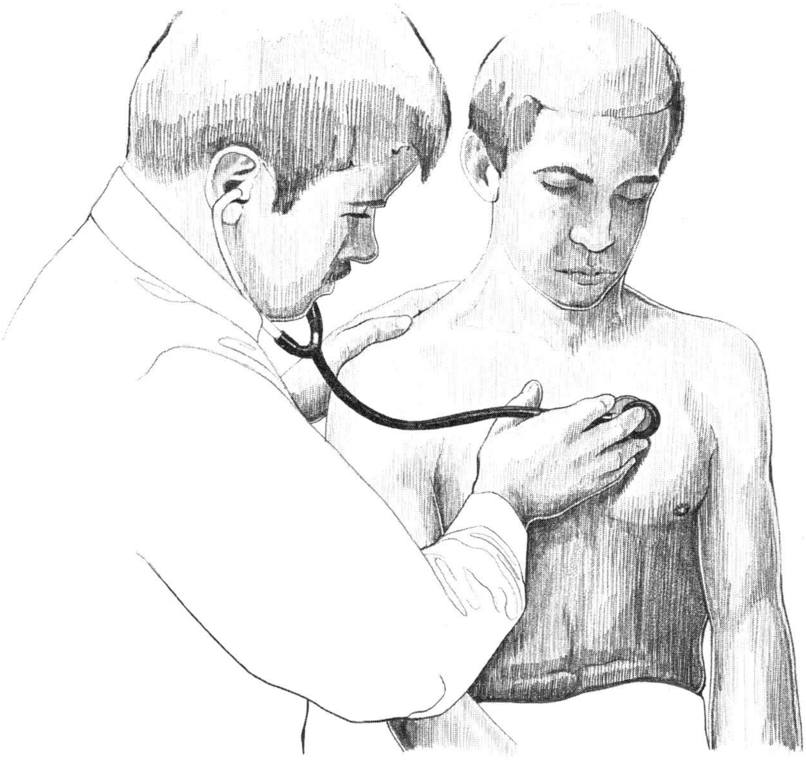

An important part of the examination of the heart is to listen for abnormal sounds and rhythm disturbances with a stethoscope.

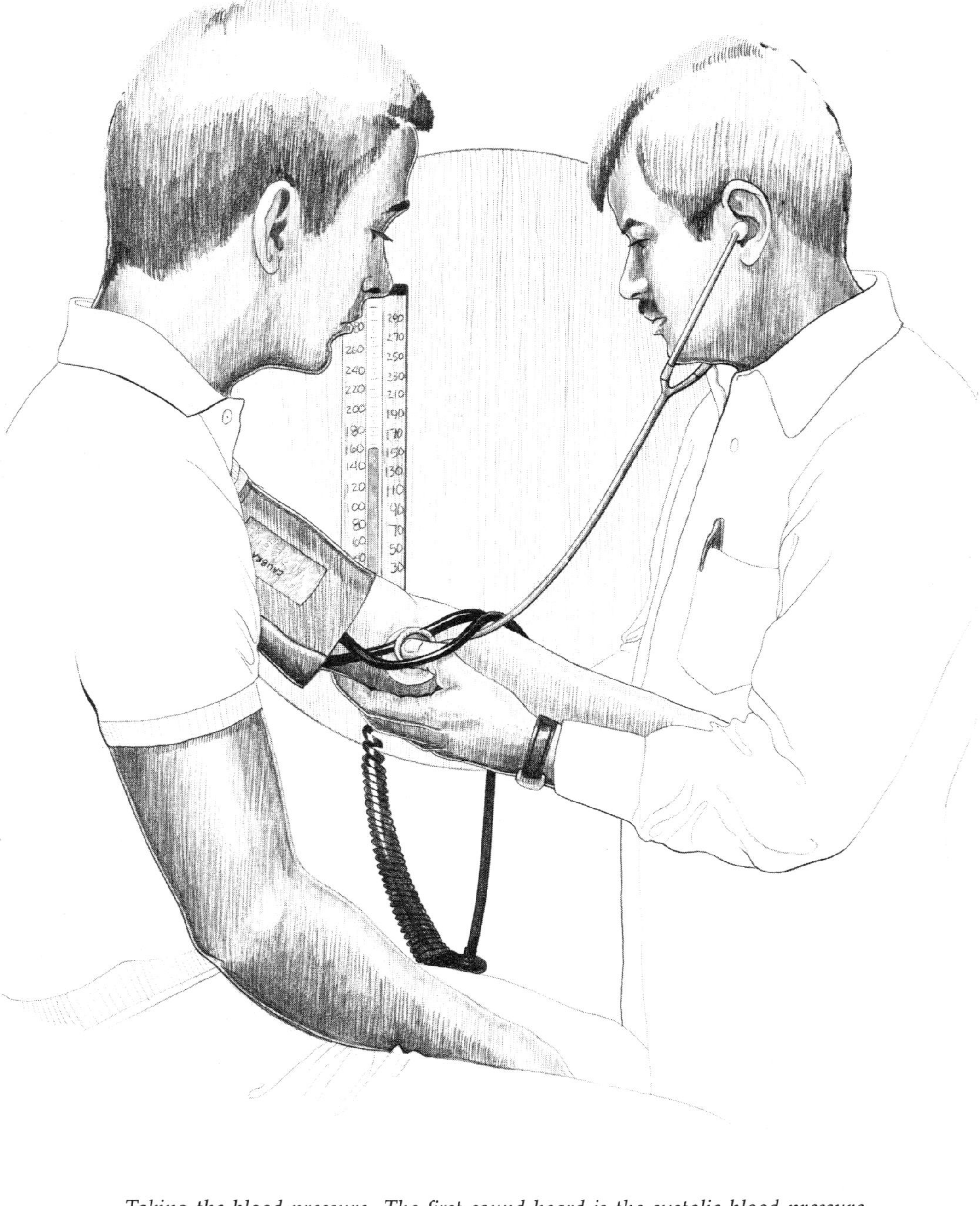

Taking the blood pressure. The first sound heard is the systolic blood pressure and the last sound is the diastolic.

The physician or technician then continues to let air out of the cuff until the cuff no longer compresses the artery and the thumping sounds disappear. At that point, the air pressure in the cuff equals the *minimum,* or diastolic, blood pressure in the artery.

Blood pressure can also be measured *directly* by means of a needle inserted into an artery. The needle is attached to an instrument that continuously records the pressure of the blood in the artery. Direct measurements of blood pressure are generally used only for research purposes. They allow medical investigators to detect rapid increases and decreases in blood pressure that might otherwise be missed.

How Blood Pressure Is Regulated

Your blood pressure is by no means constant throughout the day. It increases when your body needs more blood—for example, when you are exercising—and it decreases when your body needs less blood—such as when you are relaxing. It is lowest when you are asleep. Your blood pressure may also change after you eat, after you smoke a cigarette, when your bladder is distended, when you become excited, or when you are in pain.

Sir George Pickering, a well-known British medical investigator, likes to tell professional audiences about the marked changes in blood pressure that can occur normally. Investigators hooked up a thirty-one-year-old physician to a direct measuring device and measured his blood pressure for a 24-hour period in which he engaged in normal activities. During sexual intercourse, his blood pressure rose from 85/60 to 160/100 mm Hg. He then fell asleep and the blood pressure dropped rapidly to 60/30 mm Hg.

Such marked fluctuations in blood pressure depend on changes in the amount of blood that the heart pumps and on changes in the diameter of the arterioles. Just as increasing the amount of water that flows through a garden hose increases the water pressure in the hose, so increasing the amount of blood that the heart pumps increases the pressure in the arteries. And just as decreasing the diameter of the nozzle opening of a garden hose increases the water pressure in the hose, so decreasing the diameter of the arterioles increases the blood pressure in the arteries.

The pumping action of the heart and the diameter of the arterioles are in turn regulated by the body's chemical messengers, known as hormones, which are secreted into the blood by different organs and glands of the body and by the nervous system.

An important action of hormones is to cause the arterioles to decrease in diameter. They do this by acting on the thin layers of smooth muscle cells that ensheath each arteriole, causing it to constrict. Thus certain hormones can signal these smooth muscle cells to contract, whereas others signal them to relax. Every time the smooth muscle cells encircling the arterioles contract, the arterioles constrict. Every time these muscles relax, the arterioles expand.

Among the hormones that cause the smooth muscle cells of the arterioles to contract is norepinephrine (nor'-epp-uh-neff'-rin). This hormone is secreted as part of the body's alarm system, the so-called fight-or-flight reaction. Norepinephrine is delivered directly to the arterioles because it is released by nerves that contract the smooth muscle cells encircling the arterioles.

Hormones also affect blood pressure by altering the amount of blood that the heart pumps. The heart is largely composed of muscle. Hormones, such as norepinephrine, act on heart muscle and cause the heart to contract more strongly with each beat. The stronger contractions mean that more blood is pumped with each beat.

Hormones can also change the amount of blood that the heart pumps by altering the total volume of blood in the body. If the volume of blood increases, the heart pumps more blood and blood pressure increases. One action of renin (ree'-nin), which is a hormone made by the kidney, is to increase blood volume by causing the body to retain salt. When salt is retained, so is water; much of this extra water enters the bloodstream and increases the volume of blood in the body. Renin also causes the formation of another hormone called angiotensin, which constricts the muscle cells of the arterioles.

The nervous system also regulates the arterioles and the heart. However, not all nerves participate in this regulation; those that do are the nerves that form the *autonomic nervous*

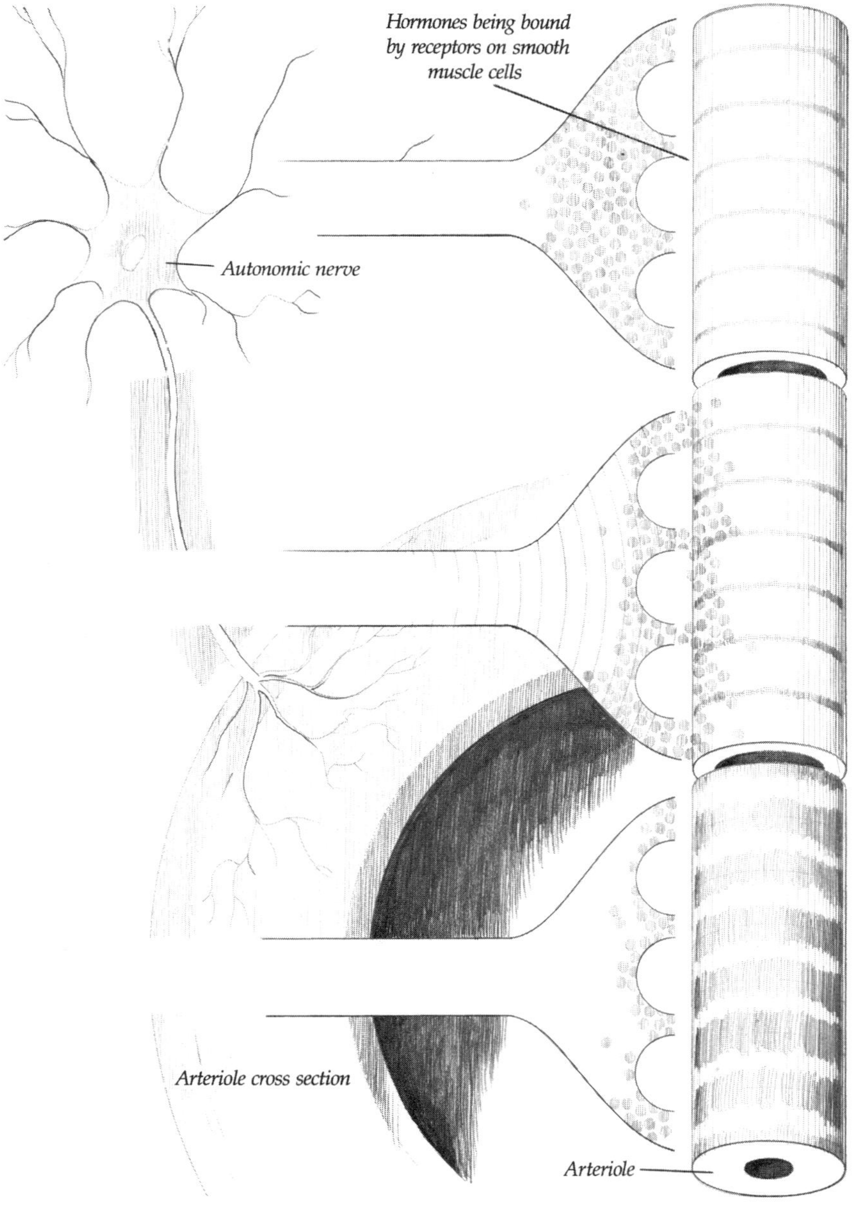

Both hormones and autonomic nerves help to regulate blood pressure. The nerves trigger the release of certain hormones, and these hormones, in turn, act on the smooth muscle cells surrounding the arterioles, causing them to contract. Other hormones cause the arterioles to relax.

system. This part of the nervous system is involuntary. Its nerves are not consciously controlled.

The autonomic nervous system is divided into two parts whose actions more or less oppose each other. The *parasympathetic* part controls bodily functions in the absence of stress. The *sympathetic* part is the body's alarm system. It speeds up the heart, increasing the amount of blood that the heart pumps and thus increasing blood pressure. It is also responsible for the release of the hormone norepinephrine, which causes arterioles to contract. In addition, it causes veins to contract, forcing blood to return to the heart more quickly, which increases the amount of blood that the heart pumps.

The Master Control System

Hormones and the nervous system act on the arterioles and the heart to make your blood pressure go up or down, depending on whether you are awake or asleep, nervous or calm. But, if you have hypertension, your blood pressure is always higher than that of a person with normal blood pressure under similar conditions.

The situation is analogous to the control of temperature in your house. Suppose that you set the thermostat for a particular temperature, say 72°F. The thermostat turns the furnace on and off so that the temperature in your house never varies much from 72°. Your neighbors may set their thermostat at 68°. The temperature in their house may, under certain conditions, reach 72° before their thermostat turns off their furnace, but, on the average, their house is cooler than yours.

In the same way, each person's blood pressure is set to fall within a particular range by a regulator, called a barostat (bahr'-oh-stat), which is similar in principle to the thermostat. (*Baro* is the Greek word for pressure.) If you have high blood pressure, your barostat is set higher than it would be if your blood pressure were normal. As a result, your physician may find it difficult to lower your blood pressure. The problem is that the barostat reacts to the lowered blood pressure as being abnormal and tries to bring it up again. Fortunately, the problem can be overcome. When the blood pressure is lowered and maintained at a lower level for a time, the barostat will adjust to this lower pressure by becoming reset. It may then be possible to decrease the dose of drugs because the reset barostat will help maintain the lower blood pressure. *However, you should never try to change your dose of drugs without your physician's permission. You may be tampering with your life.*

The barostat is composed of nerves called baroreceptors. These nerves are present in the upper part of the aorta, which is the large artery leading from the heart, and in the carotid (kuh-rah'-tid) arteries in the neck. The endings of the baroreceptor nerves are imbedded in the walls of these arteries. When blood pressure increases, the arterial expansion stretches these nerve endings. This stimulates the nerves to signal the brain to reduce the activity of the sympathetic

Baroreceptor nerve endings lie in the muscle wall of the carotid arteries, as shown here, and in the upper part of the aorta.

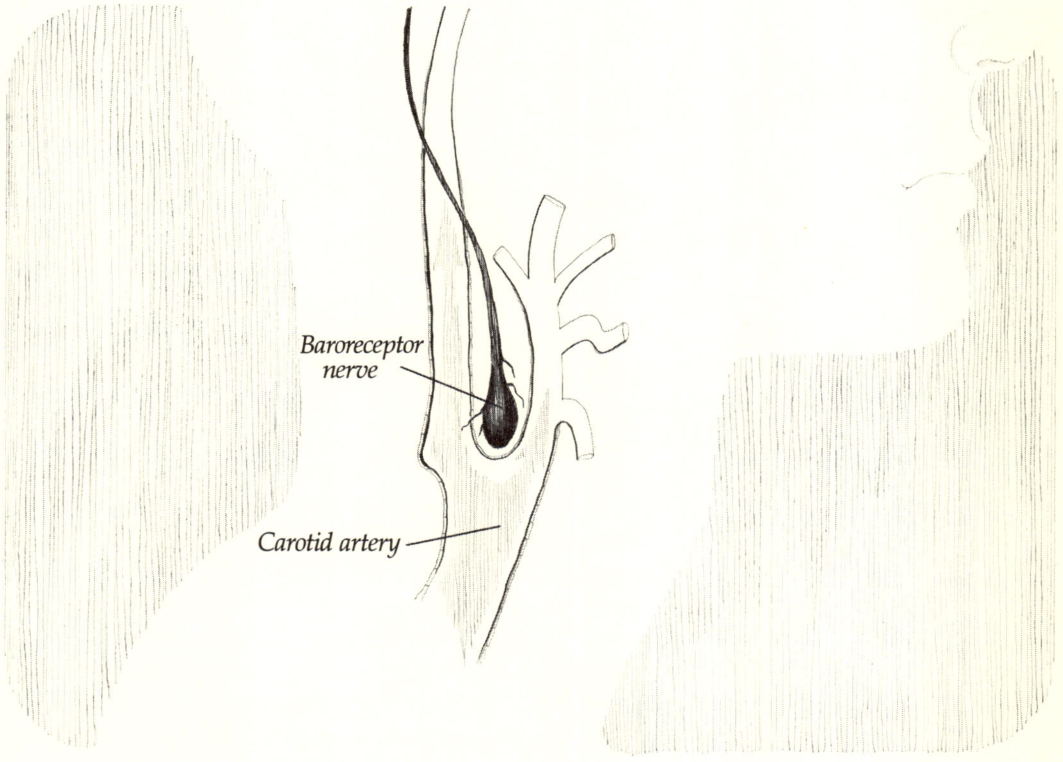

nervous system. The result is a slowing of the heart rate, a dilation of the arterioles, and a drop in blood pressure. The baroreceptor nerves can also sense when the blood pressure is too low. Then they signal the brain to stimulate the sympathetic nervous system and raise the blood pressure.

What Causes Blood Pressure to Rise?

We have already mentioned that people who have high blood pressure have barostats that are set too high. Although medical investigators do not yet know why this occurs, they do know its major effect: *The arterioles of people with high blood pressure seem to be more constricted than those of people whose blood pressure is normal.*

It is the constriction of the arterioles that causes blood pressure to rise. Blood pressure can also rise when the heart pumps more blood, but measurements of the amount of blood pumped in people with high blood pressure indicate that their hearts pump no more blood than do those of people with normal blood pressure.

When Is Blood Pressure High?

Sir George Pickering pointed out in 1955 that high blood pressure is unlike most other diseases. There is no distinct dividing line between normal and abnormal blood pressures, between those who do and those who do not have the disease.

Pickering notes that there have been numerous definitions of hypertension through the years. Among them are eight definitions that vary from classifying hypertension as blood pressures above 120/80 to classifying it as pressures above 180/110. Pickering explains, "It is clear that not all of the eight definitions can be right. Is there evidence for any? I have challenged every medical audience to whom I have spoken for twenty years to produce it. None has been forthcoming because there is none. These dividing lines are nothing more or less than artifacts."

If no one knows what the dividing line between normal and abnormal blood pressure is, how can your physician decide whether you have hypertension?

Careful studies have shown that the higher your blood pressure, the more likely you are to die or be disabled from cardiovascular diseases or strokes. It is in the light of what we know of these consequences that medical investigators agree to designate one range of blood pressures "normal" and another range "high." The ranges for normal and high blood pressures are not set in stone, but they are important guidelines. If your blood pressure is in the "high" range, there is no doubt that the risk of your dying or becoming disabled is increased—unless, of course, the blood pressure is lowered with adequate treatment.

Medical investigators agreed to call blood pressures greater than 160/95 definite hypertension. This means that, if your systolic blood pressure is greater than 160 (no matter what your diastolic pressure is), you have hypertension. Alternatively, if your diastolic pressure is greater than 95 (no matter what your systolic pressure is), you have hypertension.

Borderline hypertension is defined as blood pressures between 140/90 and 160/95. Once again, either the systolic or the diastolic blood pressure can put you in this range. A person with borderline hypertension should periodically check his blood pressure to make sure that it has not increased to the definite hypertensive category. The National Heart, Lung, and Blood Institute estimates that 25 million Americans have borderline hypertension, compared with 35 million with definite hypertension.

Finally, the definition of normal blood pressure is anything below 140/90. Contrary to what was previously thought about low blood pressure, the lower your blood pressure, the less the risk of heart attacks or strokes. However, if your blood pressure is in the normal range, the advantage of reducing it further is not great enough to justify the use of antihypertensive drugs. For people with normal blood pressures, the benefits of the drugs would not outweigh their potential risks.

CHAPTER 2

A DISEASE OF MODERN LIVING?

Most people with high blood pressure, or hypertension, have what is known as *essential hypertension,* or hypertension of unknown cause. Although it usually can be controlled with drugs, essential hypertension can only rarely be cured. Patients with essential hypertension must be treated for the rest of their lives or their blood pressures will remain high.

Essential hypertension is so common that it accounts for more than 95 percent of all cases of high blood pressure. The remaining cases are caused by definite physical abnormalities. These abnormalities can sometimes be corrected and the patients' hypertension cured.

Because the curable forms of hypertension are so rare, they will be discussed only briefly in the following chapter. In this chapter we will concentrate on what are thought to be the causes of essential hypertension.

Since nearly one out of every six Americans has essential hypertension, it must be caused by something commonplace, something nearly everyone is exposed to.

Hypertension may also be caused by something that only recently appeared in our environment because it seems to be a disease of modern living. Members of primitive societies who live the way all people did before the organization of cities and states do not have high blood pressure. In addition, unlike that of people living in industrialized societies, primitive people's blood pressure does not rise as they grow older.

By comparing life in primitive societies with life in more advanced societies, medical investigators hope to find clues to the causes of hypertension. They often cite three differences between the two ways of life: people in primitive societies are presumed to be under less stress, they have little salt in their diets, and they are not obese. *Stress, salt, and obesity have thus been suggested as causes of hypertension.*

Additional evidence implicating stress, salt, and obesity comes from experiments with human beings and with animals. Using human subjects, investigators have tried to lower blood pressure by eliminating sources of stress, by reducing their intake of salt, or by helping them to lose weight. They have also tried to develop high blood pressure in animal subjects by placing them under stress or by giving them a high-salt or high-calorie diet.

Stress

That stress is an important cause of high blood pressure is a commonly held belief in the United States. We have heard stress discussed on television and have read about it in magazines and newspapers. Many books have been published on how to relieve stress through relaxation. Many of our companies and organizations sponsor seminars and workshops on how to deal with stress. But in the medical community, opinion is divided about how important a role stress plays in hypertension and how effective relaxation can be in preventing or curing it.

There is medical evidence that implicates stress as a cause of hypertension, but this evidence is sometimes equivocal and occasionally contradictory. The same holds true for the effectiveness of relaxation techniques for curing hypertension. The lack of definitive evidence is what raises doubts in the medical community.

A common approach to determining whether a relationship exists between stress and high blood pressure is to look at the health records of large groups of people. This sounds straightforward enough, but medical investigators who carried out such experiments have come across a major obstacle: they often find that when stress is present so are other factors, such as obesity. These factors could by themselves cause high blood pressure.

Medical investigators sometimes disagree about the importance of stress relative to these other conditions. For example, some say that stress can account for the high incidences of hypertension among black Americans because being black in our society is a stressful condition. Others place more weight on other aspects of being black. Blacks may be genetically predisposed to develop hypertension. Or their hypertension may be related to their concentration in the lower socioeconomic classes. Hypertension is more common in lower socioeconomic groups, perhaps because of diet. Another explanation is that blacks, as a group, tend to be overweight in comparison with whites. There is good evidence that obese people have higher blood pressures than do those whose weight is under control.

Another type of experiment is to study stress in animals and then try to extend the conclusions to human beings. For example, animals have been subjected to stressful social conditions, such as crowding. James Henry of the School of Medicine of the University of California at Los Angeles has found that mice living in crowded cages develop high blood pressure, whereas those living in less crowded environments do not.

It is not clear, however, that people develop high blood pressure when they are crowded. Some studies show that crowded city dwellers are more likely to have high blood pressure than are people living in rural areas. Other studies show just the opposite. For example, black Americans living in cities have lower blood pressures than those living in the country.

People may inherit a tendency to become hypertensive, which then becomes manifest only when they are under constant stress. Or, it has been proposed that not only stress, but also a "hypertensive personality," which may be inherited or developed very early in life, is responsible for high blood pressure.

People with hypertensive personalities are said to be nervous, to suppress their anger, and to be "tenderminded," meaning that their feelings are easily hurt. Although there is support in the medical community for the concept of hypertensive personality, not everyone has observed these traits in hypertensive patients. And not everyone believes that patients with these traits develop high blood pressure because of them.

Herbert Benson of the Harvard Medical School, who is a well-known researcher of stress, believes there is no such thing as a hypertensive personality. He points out that so-called hypertensive traits may have developed as an effect, rather than a cause, of high blood pressure. For example, patients may become nervous *after* they find out that they have high blood pressure. However, this possibility has not generally been considered, given that nearly all investigators studying personality traits look only at patients who already have high blood pressure.

Many medical investigators study the relationship between stress and high blood pressure by teaching patients biofeedback or relaxation techniques, such as transcendental meditation and yoga. The patients using these techniques presumably learn to cope with stress. Thus, if stress is a cause of high blood pressure, patients who relax may find that their blood pressures go down.

Nearly all of the studies of the effects of relaxation on blood pressure have a fundamental drawback: they do not include a group of patients (controls) who, for purposes of comparison, do not employ these techniques. It is possible that the patients' blood pressures went down merely because they became used to having their blood pressures taken or because of the power of suggestion that the behavioral techniques would help.

A good example of the strong, but temporary, effects of the power of suggestion on blood pressure can be found in an experiment that dates back to 1955. In this experiment, a dramatic-looking device was shown to a group of patients who had high blood pressure. The patients were told that the device was a "therapeutic electron gun" that would reduce their blood pressures. In fact, the device did nothing.

The systolic blood pressures of the patients "treated" with the therapeutic electron gun fell an average of 20 mm Hg. Their diastolic blood pressures fell an average of 14 mm Hg. This effect lasted several weeks, but then their blood pressures went back up. The effect of the therapeutic electron gun was similar to the effects often attributed to biofeedback and relaxation techniques.

One of the few studies of the effects of behavioral techniques on blood pressure that did include a control group of patients was conducted by a team of physicians at the National Heart, Lung, and Blood Institute. These physicians divided hypertensive patients into three groups. One group was taught relaxation and biofeedback. The second group of patients monitored their blood pressures with a biofeedback machine that gave false information. Ordinarily, a red light on the machine flashes if a person's blood pressure goes up, a yellow light flashes if it stays the same, and a green light flashes if it goes down. With the machine used by the second group of patients, the color of the light bore no relation to the changes in a patient's blood pressure. The third group of patients in this study was given no instruction on relaxation techniques or biofeedback.

The results were disappointing to the physicians conducting the study. Except for one patient in the first group whose blood pressure decreased, the blood pressures of patients in all three groups were the same after the study as before it.

There is no question, however, that stress raises blood pressure temporarily while a person is in a state of emotional excitement. Strong emotions excite the sympathetic nervous system, which causes the blood pressure to rise. When we relax and especially when we fall asleep, the sympathetic nervous system becomes inactive and the blood pressure falls. But these fluctuations in blood pressure are only temporary; such changes in a person's state do not raise the general level of blood pressure above normal, which is what happens in essential hypertension. For example, when American soldiers were being heavily bombarded at the Anzio beachhead in World War II, they were found to have high blood pressures. After the siege was over, however, their blood pressures promptly fell to normal. Obviously, they did not have essential hypertension. Rather, their sympathetic nervous systems were temporarily overactive, and this was stimulated by fear. Although we know that stress plays an important part in causing peaks of pressure in the fluctuations of blood pressure that occur throughout the day, we have no convincing evidence that this can lead to a *permanent increase* in the general level of blood pressure.

Salt (Sodium)

Deep in the jungles of western Brazil there lives a tribe of Indians called the Yanomamos. Because they are protected from the outside world by the Brazilian government, the Yanomamos continue to live as they have done for thousands of years. The Yanomamos are a healthy and spirited race. They have been called the "fierce people" because of constant warfare between the villages.

Several years ago, William Oliver of the University of Michigan obtained permission from the Brazilian government to study the Yanomamos in their native habitat. Oliver and a team of researchers set up camp in one of the villages. They were there for many months travelling from village to village and studying not only the health of the Indians, but also their culture and habits. Of greatest interest to us are their observations on hypertension—or rather the lack of it. In about 1,000 natives examined, they found not a single case of high blood pressure. To realize what this means, we should tell you that in the same number of Americans more than 125 hypertensives would be detected. Also, in our society blood pressure slowly rises as we grow older. Not so with the Yanomamos. The elderly members of the tribe exhibited the same low normal levels of blood pressure as did the youngsters.

The maintenance of a low normal blood pressure throughout life without hypertension is not limited to the Yanomamo Indians. As we have already mentioned, hypertension has been found to be absent in other peoples who were isolated from the modern world and living under primitive conditions, such as in certain of the South Sea Islands and in remote parts of Africa.

These primitive tribes must have something in common that prevents them from developing hypertension. The first thought that comes to most of us is that they are spared hypertension because they are not exposed to the stress and the fast pace of modern living. But this explanation does not hold up very well on close examination. As already noted in this chapter, the evidence implicating stress as a cause of hypertension is pretty weak. For example, blood pressure has been measured only since the turn of the century but, if we consider the pace of living in the first quarter of this century to have been slower than it is now, we should expect that hypertension was less common then compared with the present. Although exact comparisons are not possible because records in those days were less complete, we know that hypertension was a common condition then. One more thought. Primitive people have their stresses too. Food sources are often uncertain. The elements can be punishing, and their culture is filled with taboos and superstitions. In fact, the Yanomamos are in a constant state of war.

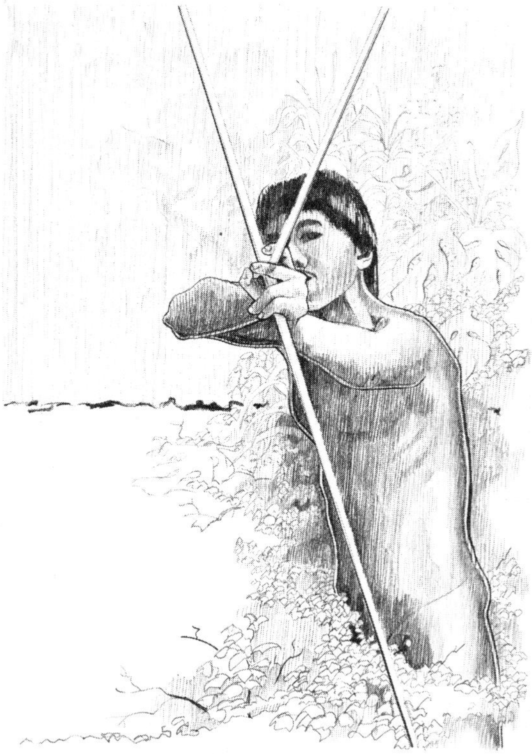

If not a lack of stress, what other aspects of primitive civilization could prevent hypertension? Oliver cast about for an explanation and then he made a most striking discovery. To his surprise, he found almost no sodium in the urine of the Yanomamos—in fact, less than one percent of what we excrete. The amount of sodium voided in the urine indicates fairly accurately the amount we take in through diet. The observation meant that the Yanomamos eat only a fraction of the sodium that we do.

We have many sources of sodium in our diet in addition to common table salt, or sodium chloride. Even those of us who don't salt our food still eat an excess of sodium because sodium chloride or other sodium compounds have already been added to the foods we buy in the market. All canned foods, baked goods, smoked meats, and many dairy products contain added sodium. Snack foods are loaded with it. The average American consumes about 3,000 to 6,000 milligrams of sodium per day, most of it added by the food industry to the products that we eat. One level teaspoon of salt, for example, contains about 2,300 milligrams of sodium. A slice of American cheese contains about 890 milligrams of sodium. Even when we try to limit our salt intake, the best we can do is to reduce it to about 1,500 milligrams of sodium per day, which is still *fifty times as much as* the amount consumed by the Yanomamo Indians in a 24-hour period.

What do the Yanomamos eat? Mostly fruits, including bananas and palm fruits, wild game, and starchy roots, such as plantain. Living far inland and being isolated from the rest of the world, they have no access to salt.

Other physician-epidemiologists working in other parts of the world who have studied this problem have found evidence that strongly supports the no-salt theory. Lot Page of Boston studied six different native groups in the Solomon Islands. Three of the island groups were isolated, whereas the other three had frequent contacts with civilization. Hypertension was rare or absent in the three isolated islands but was present in the others. Page found that the frequency with which he detected hypertension in each group correlated with the amount of sodium he found in their urine: the greater the sodium excretion, the higher the incidence of hypertension.

Frank Lowenstein, a Brazilian physician, studied two native tribes, the Carajos and the Munducurus in the Amazon river basin. The Munducurus had been converted by missionaries who also habituated the tribe to the use of table salt. Lowenstein found that hypertension was common among the Mundurucus and was absent among the Carajos.

These observations and many others strongly suggest that salt, or more precisely sodium, is the culprit in the appearance of hypertension as a disease of civilized man. But such studies cannot supply final proof. The only way to obtain such evidence would be to feed salt to the native populations without changing their life style in any other way. If the theory is correct, the blood pressure should rise. This experiment has never been done because the epidemiologists did not consider it ethical.

There are, however, other lines of evidence that relate sodium to hypertension more directly. One of them was provided by a refugee from the Nazis, Walter Kempner, a physician who settled in Durham, North Carolina, in the early 1940s. Kempner had the idea that hypertension was due to a defect in the excretion of protein waste products and sodium by the kidney. He reasoned that, if protein and sodium were eliminated from the diet, the defective kidney would be put at rest and the hypertension would improve. Kempner devised a diet that consisted only of rice, fruit, sugar, and vitamin tablets. Nothing else was permitted. He required that the patients remain on the diet for one hundred days and, to insure that his instructions were followed, he established "rice-houses" in Durham where the patients were required to stay until the hundred days were up.

Because the diet was so strict, only those patients whose hypertension was the most severe and complicated would accept it. Many of these patients had heart and kidney damage, often with uremic poisoning. Unlikely as it may seem, the treatment was successful. The blood pressures of many of the patients decreased markedly, and their general health improved.

It was not long afterward that other researchers determined that it was the absence of sodium rather than the low protein content of the diet that brought about the decrease in blood pressure. They showed that the addition of about 500 milligrams of sodium to the rice diet caused the blood pressure to rise again, an amount that is only about one-tenth that of the sodium we normally eat.

The results of the rice-and-fruit diet and the studies of primitive peoples indicate that human beings can live a healthy life with a very low intake of sodium. On the other hand, human beings, like other animals, crave salt. We know that salt was highly valued in ancient times. Roman soldiers, for example, were often paid in salt and the word "salary" comes from this custom. The phrase "A man is worth his salt" indicates the value placed on salt since olden times. In the days of the feudal lords, guests took their places at the dinner table according to rank and favor. Their positions at the table were determined by the location of the salt dispenser, those of highest rank sitting "with the salt" and the lesser lights seating themselves "beneath the salt."

Why has salt been valued so highly throughout the history of civilization? Why do animals travel many miles to reach a salt lick? We do not know. Primitive people can get along without salt with no loss of health or strength. The Kalahari Bushmen of South Africa trek across the hot desert in pursuit of game for many miles despite a very low salt

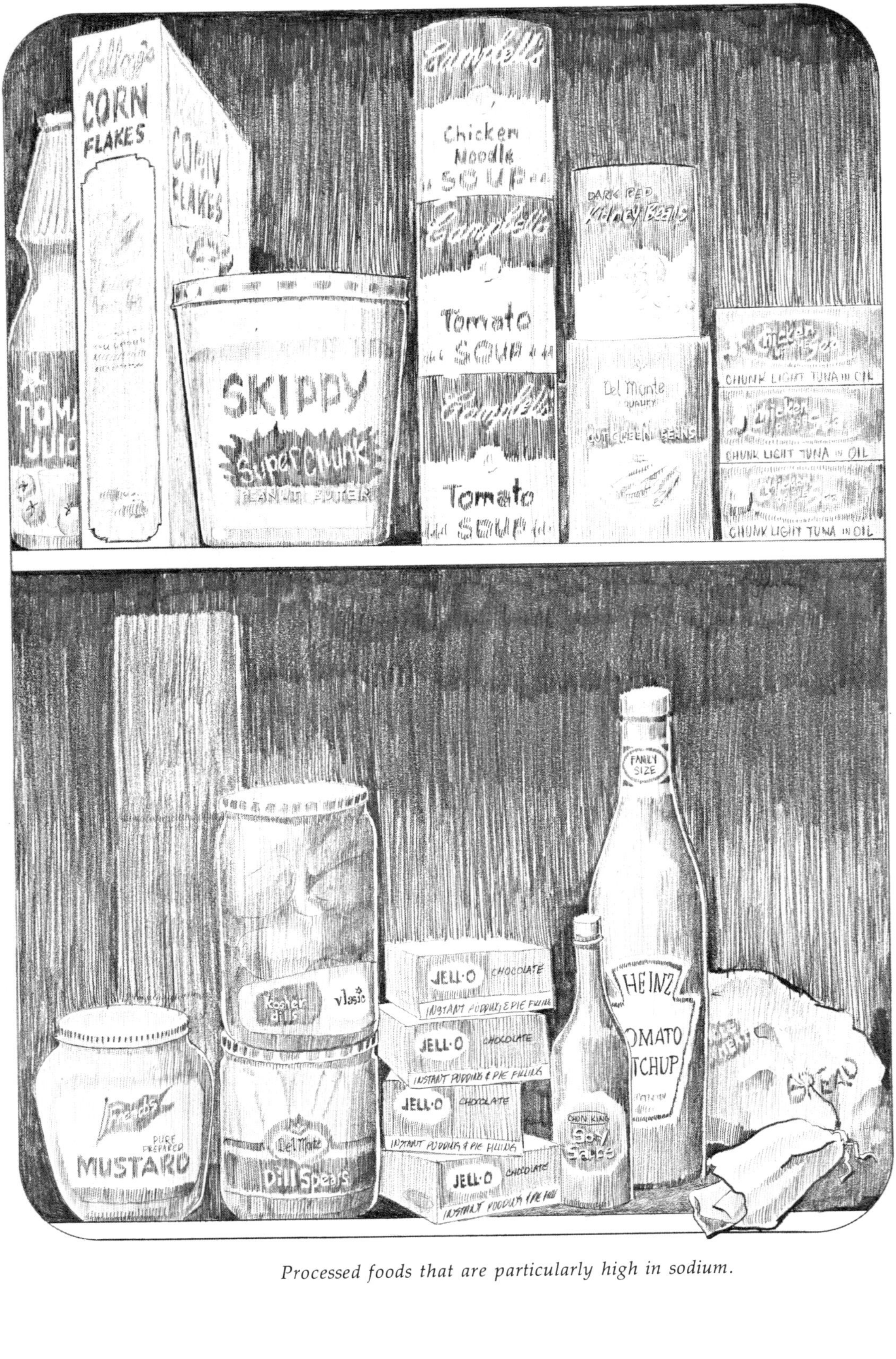

Processed foods that are particularly high in sodium.

intake. Although the cause of the salt addiction is unknown, it is apparent that beyond a bare minimum salt is not needed for our continued good health.

Strict low-sodium diets such as the rice-and-fruit diet are rarely prescribed today because their monotony and unpalatability make them intolerable. The thiazide diuretic drugs that became available in 1958 have replaced strict low-sodium diets. When taken continuously, these drugs reduce body sodium and lower blood pressure by the same amount as did the rice-and-fruit diet.

Is there still a place for low-sodium diets in the treatment of hypertension? Diets that are moderately low in sodium (that is, those in which normal intake is reduced by one-half or two-thirds) are much more palatable than the rice-and-fruit diet, but they are usually effective only to a degree. For example, a group of Belgian physicians prescribed a diet that excluded foods high in sodium but permitted other foods such as fresh meats, vegetables, and fruits. Lemon juice was used as a salt substitute. The blood pressure of patients who followed this diet fell moderately but not to the degree that can be obtained with the thiazide diuretics.

Nevertheless, given the fact that sodium consumption has increased through the centuries beyond all bounds intended by nature, it is difficult to deny that it could well be harmful. In the United States, the average daily sodium consumption has increased from about 2,400 milligrams to 3,600 milligrams in a single generation. This is due to the enthusiasm of the food-processing industry, which continues to add more and more sodium in the form of table salt and other sodium compounds to our foods, particularly to snack foods.

In this connection, it should be noted that the taste buds become adjusted to the saltiness of food. When heavily salted food is eaten, the sensitivity of the taste buds to salt becomes blunted. On the contrary, when the diet is low in salt, they become quite sensitive so that even a modest amount of salt is unpalatable. If we are heavy salt eaters, we require more and more salt because of the loss of sensitivity of the taste buds, which may be one reason that the food processors add such large amounts to certain foods. If our salt intake were reduced, our taste buds would adjust in a week or two so that much smaller amounts of salt in our food would produce a salty flavor.

Can any of the salt substitutes available in drug stores and supermarkets be used? Yes, but most of them are mixtures of sodium and potassium salts. Some of them contain as much as 50 percent sodium salts. So, read the labels carefully and select the one that contains the least amount of sodium. Or better yet, don't use a salt substitute at all; instead, use lemon juice, which does not contain sodium, to flavor your food.

We believe that the increasing amounts of sodium added in the form of table salt to processed foods should be halted and their sodium content should be gradually reduced. If this is not possible, then at least the sodium content should be clearly stated on the label and low-sodium items should be more readily available. Appendix A gives the sodium content of many of the foodstuffs you buy in the supermarket. We hope that you will become familiar with it. There is today enough evidence to indicate that sodium is a major factor in producing hypertension in susceptible persons: that is, those who have a definite family history of hypertension or young persons who have transient periods of high blood pressure. Given our present knowledge, reducing the consumption of sodium seems to be an eminently sensible thing to do in order to prevent the development of high blood pressure in the future. For those who already have established hypertension, sodium restriction may not be sufficient to adequately control blood pressure, but it is still a useful adjunct that may reduce the amount of drug treatment that would otherwise be needed.

Obesity

For years, physicians have been reporting that overweight people are more likely to develop hypertension than are people of normal weight. They also report that, when obese people lose weight, their blood pressures drop.

Yet many physicians have soft-pedaled recommmendations that obese patients with high blood pressure lose weight. These physicians do not question the evidence that ties obesity to hypertension. This evidence is well established and convincing. For example, no one doubts the conclusions of the Framingham Study, which was a study of heart disease and high blood pressure in adults living in the town of Framingham, Massachusetts. Medical investigators found that Framingham men who lost 15 percent of their weight had a 10 percent drop in their systolic blood pressures. Those who gained 15 percent in weight gained 18 percent in their systolic blood pressures.

Why, then, haven't all physicians recommended that overweight patients with high blood pressure reduce? The answer goes back to a widespread belief in the medical community that the reason obese people have high blood pressure is that, when they eat a lot of food, they also consume a lot of sodium. When these people diet, they reduce their sodium consumption. It is the decrease in sodium intake and not the decrease in weight that causes their blood pressures to come down. According to this belief, overweight people could reduce their blood pressures just as well if they stayed obese but cut down on sodium or used drugs to rid their bodies of excess sodium and water.

One reason for the belief that the true culprit is sodium rather than obesity is that the findings of a study conducted by the late Lewis Dahl, a physician at Brookhaven Laboratory, have long supported it. Dahl put eight overweight hypertensive patients in the hospital. He gave half of them a low-calorie diet but did not reduce their sodium consumption. He gave the others a low-sodium diet but did not reduce the number of calories they consumed. The result was that the blood pressures of the patients on the low-sodium diet fell. But only two of the patients on the low-calorie diet had a reduction in blood pressure.

A number of physicians who believed in this sodium theory are now revising their opinions, partly because of the results of a much larger study conducted in Israel. A group of Israeli physicians recruited 121 overweight patients with hypertension. They encouraged 95 of these patients to lose weight but to follow a balanced diet and to eat plenty of low-calorie foods, including salty foods. The remaining 26 patients were not instructed to lose weight or change their sodium consumption.

The patients advised to lose weight lost an average of 22 pounds during the two-month study. Their blood pressures fell dramatically, even though their sodium consumption did not decrease. Most of these patients' blood pressures came down from the hypertensive to the normal range. In contrast, blood pressures remained high in the 26 patients who did not lose weight.

The Israeli study has changed the opinion of the medical profession. *Many authorities now believe that reducing diets are the best method, other than drugs, for controlling blood pressure.*

CHAPTER 3

RARE CAUSES OF HIGH BLOOD PRESSURE

Of the 35 million Americans who have high blood pressure, less than five percent have the disease because of a known physical disorder. The disorders responsible in most cases are those of the kidney, the adrenal gland, and the large artery leading out of the heart. Although hypertension thus caused is every bit as dangerous as essential hypertension, the disorder can be corrected in some cases and the high blood pressure cured.

Kidney Disorders

Damage to the arteries of the kidneys is the most common *known* cause of high blood pressure. In this form of hypertension, called renal hypertension, the arteries are narrowed because of disease and the flow of blood through the kidneys is reduced. When this happens, the kidneys release the hormone renin, which causes the blood pressure to rise. The increase in blood pressure forces more blood to flow through the narrowed arteries of the kidneys. Thus, the kidneys have a built-in feedback mechanism for restoring the blood flow in the kidney to normal. However, it does so by causing hypertension in the rest of the body.

Most people whose high blood pressure is due to kidney damage have had a disease called glomerulonephritis (glah'-mair-yuh-low-ni-fright'-us). This disease is caused by a reaction to an infection due to streptococcal bacteria anywhere in the body. The body fights these bacteria by producing antibodies that attach themselves to the bacterial invaders and destroy them. However, in some people, antibodies are produced that cross-react with kidney cells and damage them, resulting in glomerulonephritis. The damage slowly progresses over the years, affecting the small arteries throughout the kidneys. The arteries become scarred and narrowed and blood flow is reduced. This stimulates the secretion of renin by the kidneys and the patient eventually develops high blood pressure. This form of high blood pressure can often be treated with drugs. We want to emphasize that glomerulonephritis is a rare disease. Most people who get strep throats or other streptococcal infections recover completely and never develop glomerulonephritis.

Blood flow through a kidney can also be reduced when a main artery leading to the kidney is obstructed. In older patients, obstructions are almost always due to atherosclerotic plaques in kidney arteries. These plaques, which consist partly of fats and cholesterol, slowly build up in the arteries as people age. An obstructed kidney artery also is a possible cause of hypertension in the young, especially young women aged twenty to thirty-five. In some cases, the obstruction is caused by a peculiar thickening that seems to be due to

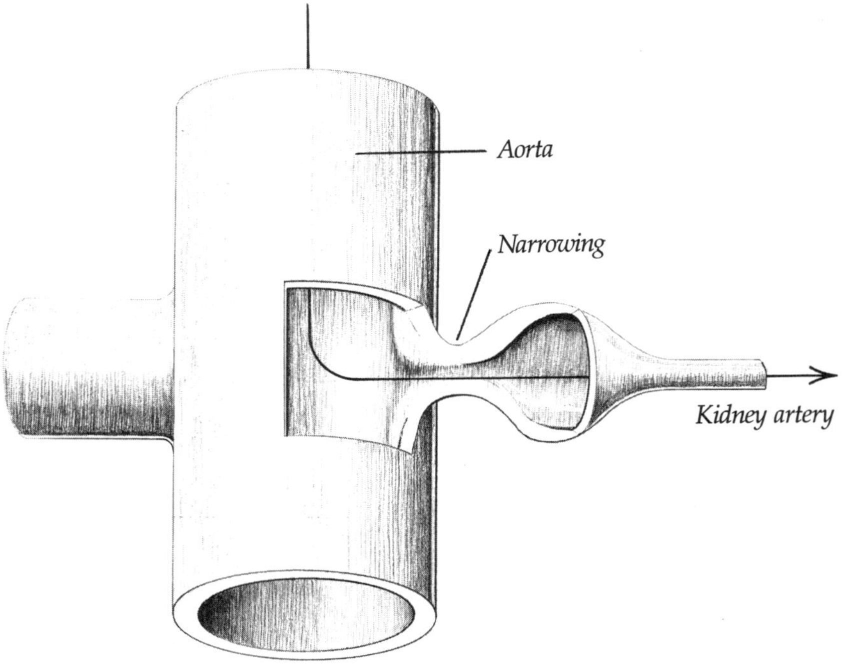

Obstructed kidney artery.

inflammation, although no evidence of infection is found. We do not know why this thickening occurs or why young women are most likely to develop it.

A physician may suspect blocked kidney arteries if the patient is a young woman with unexplained hypertension or an older person who suddenly develops severe hypertension. To help diagnose obstructions of the kidney arteries, the physician will use a stethoscope to listen to the sounds produced in the patient's abdomen. A high-pitched murmur could be an indication of a narrowed kidney artery. If the physician strongly suspects this, a search for the obstruction may be made by means of an arteriogram or a pyelogram, which are specific types of x-ray photographs. To obtain these photographs, a radiologist first injects a dye into the patient's bloodstream. The dye absorbs x-rays and allows the flow of blood through the kidney arteries to be seen in the arteriogram or pyelogram. The dye is excreted by the kidneys.

At the same time as the radiologist x-rays the patient's kidneys, he measures the output of the hormone renin by the kidneys. This is done by threading a catheter up from a vein in a leg into the main vein draining each kidney. The amount of renin found in the blood coming from each kidney is then determined. This measurement is made because not everyone with an obstructed kidney artery develops hypertension. However, if the affected kidney is producing large amounts of renin, as measured from the blood samples, the patient's high blood pressure is probably caused by the obstruction.

When an obstructed kidney artery is discovered in a young patient, the physician may refer that patient to a surgeon for removal of the obstructed part or for the implantation of an artificial blood vessel to shunt blood past the obstruction. Surgery is not so successful in older people whose kidney arteries tend to be clogged by atherosclerotic plaques. These people are usually treated with drugs.

Adrenal Disorders

Other hormones besides the kidney hormone renin cause blood pressure to rise. Among them are several hormones secreted by the adrenal glands, which are situated just above the kidneys.

Some patients have adrenal tumors that cause these glands to overproduce one of the pressure-raising hormones. Other patients have disorders that cause hormone-producing adrenal cells to be overstimulated and to produce too much hormone. In either case, the effect is the same—an overproduction of hormone—and the result is hypertension.

Aldosteronism. One of the adrenal hormones that raises blood pressure is aldosterone (al-dah'-stair-own). This hormone causes the body to retain sodium, an action that increases blood volume and also blood pressure. *Oversecretion of aldosterone is a disorder known as aldosteronism.*

The typical patient with aldosteronism is a woman between the ages of 35 and 50. Her symptoms are muscular weakness, excessive thirst, and excessive urination.

Physicians suspect aldosteronism when they find a low level of potassium in the blood. They diagnose aldosteronism by looking for three distinctive chemical abnormalities in their patients' blood and urine. Patients with this disorder have high concentrations of aldosterone in their blood because of their overactive aldosterone-producing cells. They also have low concentrations of the kidney hormone renin in their blood. This is because an excess of aldosterone in the blood inhibits the production of renin by the kidney. Finally, these patients have excessive amounts of potassium in their urine because aldosterone also acts on kidney cells to increase the excretion of potassium in the urine and lower the level in the blood.

When aldosteronism is caused by a tumor, the cure is to remove the tumor. When it is caused by a general overgrowth of adrenal cells that produce aldosterone, the treatment is by means of the drug spironolactone (spy-roh'-no-lack-tone). This drug specifically blocks the actions of aldosterone.

Cushing's Syndrome. Another adrenal hormone that causes sodium to be retained is cortisol (core'-ti-sahl). Like that of aldosterone, the overproduction of cortisol can cause high blood pressure. *Patients whose adrenal glands produce too much cortisol are said to have Cushing's syndrome.*

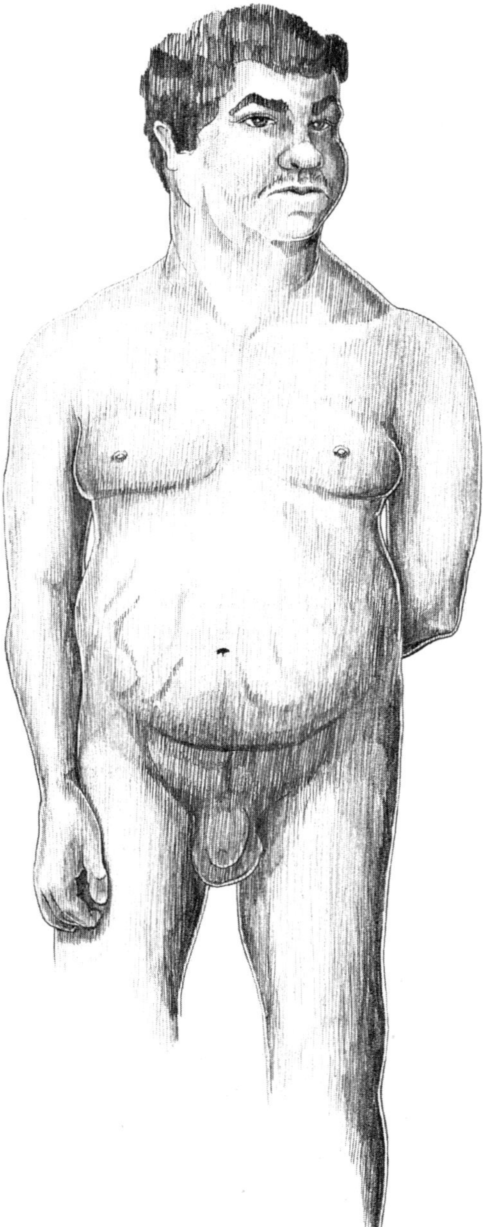

Among the characteristics of Cushing's syndrome are a round, red face, an obese body, and a pendulous belly.

The typical patient with Cushing's syndrome is easy to identify. The patient is almost always a woman, and the syndrome causes her to have a rather characteristic and often bizarre appearance. She has a round, red face, facial hair, thin scalp hair, an obese body, and a pendulous belly with purple stretch marks on it. She may have menstrual disturbances and she may be infertile. X-ray examination will reveal that her bones have too little calcium.

A physician's suspicion that a patient has Cushing's syndrome is confirmed if that patient's urine contains large amounts of cortisol. There are two treatments for Cushing's syndrome. One is to try to prevent overstimulation of the adrenal cells by irradiating the pituitary gland. This gland, which is at the base of the brain, signals the adrenal cells to produce cortisol. The second treatment is to remove both adrenal glands or all of one gland and nine-tenths of the other. Total removal is the surer treatment, but it requires life-long medication with oral hormones to replace those normally produced by the adrenals.

Pheochromocytoma. Other adrenal hormones that raise blood pressure are epinephrine (formerly called adrenaline) and norepinephrine. These hormones are secreted by a group of adrenal cells called chromaffin (crow'-muh-fin) cells. *Patients with chromaffin cell tumors, which oversecrete epinephrine and norepinephrine, have pheochromocytoma* (fee-oh-crow'-moh-sigh-toe'-muh).

This disorder is sometimes misdiagnosed. Its symptoms can mimic those of hyperthyroidism, which is due to an overactive thyroid gland. The symptoms include pounding of the heart, headache, sweating, and pale, cold skin. The patients are almost always thin.

Some patients with pheochromocytoma believe that they have a psychological disturbance. The tumors of their chromaffin cells secrete epinephrine and norepinephrine intermittently, causing their symptoms to come and go. Because the symptoms are like those of fear or alarm, the patients say that they have "fits" that come upon them suddenly. Other patients have a rapid pulse and flushed skin that mimics an overactive thyroid.

Pheochromocytoma can cause severe elevations of blood pressure—as high as 300/180 mm Hg. Physicians diagnose this disorder by testing their patients' urine. Patients who have the disorder have increased amounts of epinephrine and norepinephrine in their urine. The disease is cured by surgical removal of the tumors that produce the excess hormones.

Coarctation of the Aorta

A few people are born with a constriction of the aorta, the large artery that leaves the heart. This disorder, which causes a distinctive type of high blood pressure, is called *coarctation of the aorta*.

Because the aorta is narrowed by the constriction, the heart must pump more forcefully to get blood past the constriction and into the rest of the body. This forceful pumping of the heart causes the increased blood pressure. Because of the location of the constriction, patients have high blood

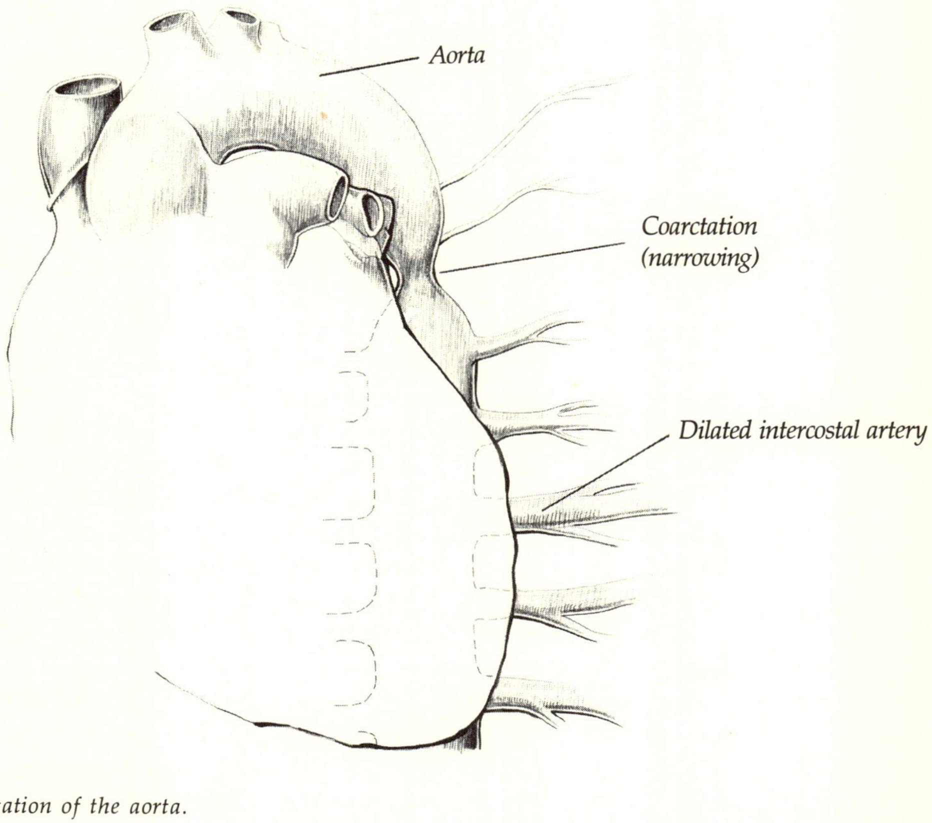

Coarctation of the aorta.

pressure in the arteries of their arms but lower blood pressure than normal in the arteries of their legs.

Coarctation of the aorta in an inherited defect that is present from birth. Because high blood pressure caused by coarctation can be recognized in childhood, we feel that it is important to measure blood pressure as a matter of course when children undergo school health examinations. If hypertension caused by coarctation is discovered in a child, the constriction of the aorta can be surgically repaired and the hypertension cured.

CHAPTER 4

WHY HIGH BLOOD PRESSURE IS DANGEROUS

Today, the medical profession is unanimous in its belief that all high blood pressure has very serious medical consequences. Acceptance of this belief, however, was slow in coming.

As recently as the early 1960s, most physicians believed that high blood pressure, unless very severe, was not harmful and in some cases was actually beneficial. They reasoned that, because the blood vessels of older people are narrower than those of younger people, older people require a high blood pressure to push blood through their vessels. If a person's blood pressure did not rise with age, the flow of blood through vital body organs would be inadequate. Physicians thought that only severe hypertension, in which the diastolic pressure is greater than 115, was dangerous.

It may seem strange that long before 1960 evidence had been obtained showing that all hypertension is dangerous. As early as 1928, the American Society of Actuaries published a report showing that people with even mild elevations of blood pressure were likely to die at earlier ages than those with normal blood pressures. Furthermore, the risk of dying increased in proportion to the height of the blood pressure. But most physicians dismissed this evidence, saying that the insurance examiners reported the blood pressures lower than they actually were so that the applicants could get insurance.

The attitude of the medical profession began to change in the early 1960s when the results of the Framingham study became known. This study is so important that it is still the most widely cited source of data on the effects of hypertension. The results of the Framingham study have since been confirmed by numerous other studies.

Because it was the Framingham results that finally convinced physicians that high blood pressure is dangerous, we will begin this section by explaining how the results were obtained. Later in the chapter we will discuss the results and relate them to the dangerous effects of high blood pressure.

The Framingham Study

The town of Framingham, Massachusetts, is an industrial and trading center about twenty miles from Boston. The Framingham study began in 1949 when about 5,000 healthy residents of the town agreed to participate in a unique long-term experiment. Medical investigators, sponsored by the National Institutes of Health, wanted to follow these people for decades, examining them for evidence of cardiovascular diseases.

Every two years, these residents of Framingham go to a special clinic for a medical examination. At the clinic, their blood chemistries (including blood cholesterol) are checked, their blood pressures are determined, and they are weighed. They have electrocardiograms taken, which indicate how their hearts function. They are also questioned about such things as their smoking, eating, and sleeping habits and about how physically active they are.

The physicians conducting the Framingham study soon had a collection of medical data unlike any that had ever before been obtained. They had complete medical records of a large group of initially healthy people, some of whom eventually had high blood pressure, strokes, heart attacks, and other cardiovascular diseases. From these records, the investigators could see whether cardiovascular diseases strike at random or whether there are clues in peoples' life-styles or medical histories that are predictive of who will get these diseases and who will not.

When they analyzed the data, the investigators discovered that people with certain traits or habits are more likely than others to develop cardiovascular diseases. They called these traits and habits risk factors. Among them were cigarette smoking, increased amounts of cholesterol in the blood, and high blood pressure. The most important was hypertension because it was a leading risk factor not only for heart attacks, but also for heart failure, strokes, and kidney damage.

THE FRAMINGHAM STUDY

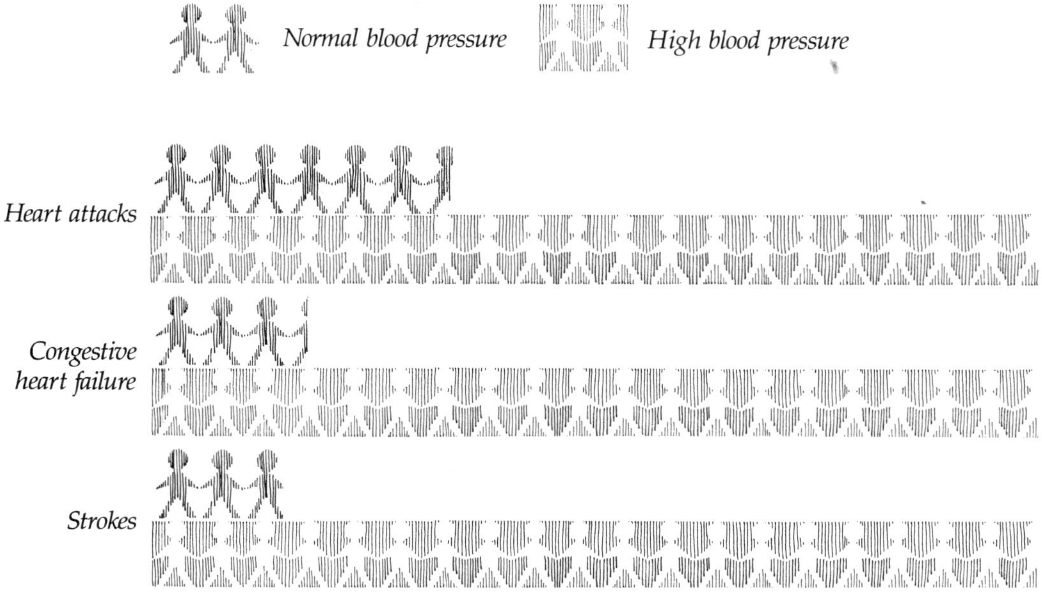

In the Framingham study, 5,209 residents between the ages of thirty-five and seventy-four underwent examination and observation for twelve years. People with hypertension had three times as many heart attacks, six times as much congestive heart failure, and seven times as many strokes as did people whose blood pressures were normal.

HIGH BLOOD PRESSURE AND HEART ATTACKS

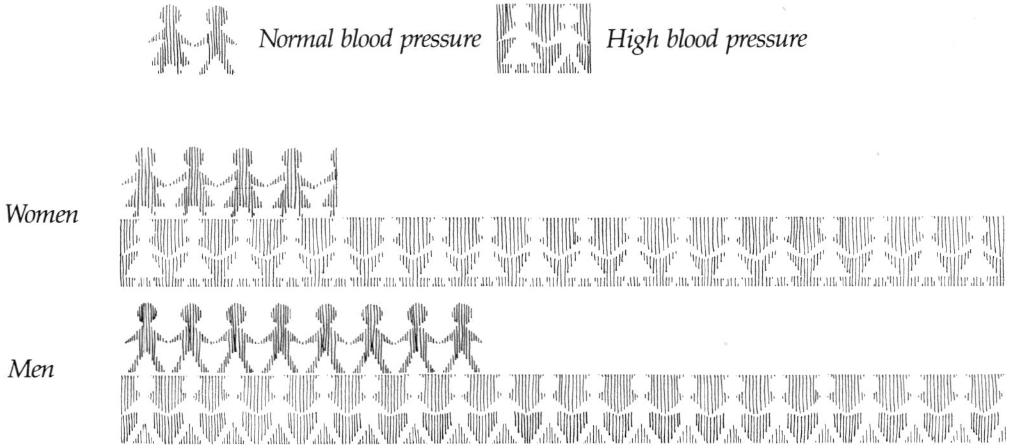

Results from the Framingham study showed that women who have hypertension are more than four times as likely to have heart attacks as are those with normal blood pressures. Men having hypertension are two and one-half times as likely to have them as are those whose blood pressures are normal.

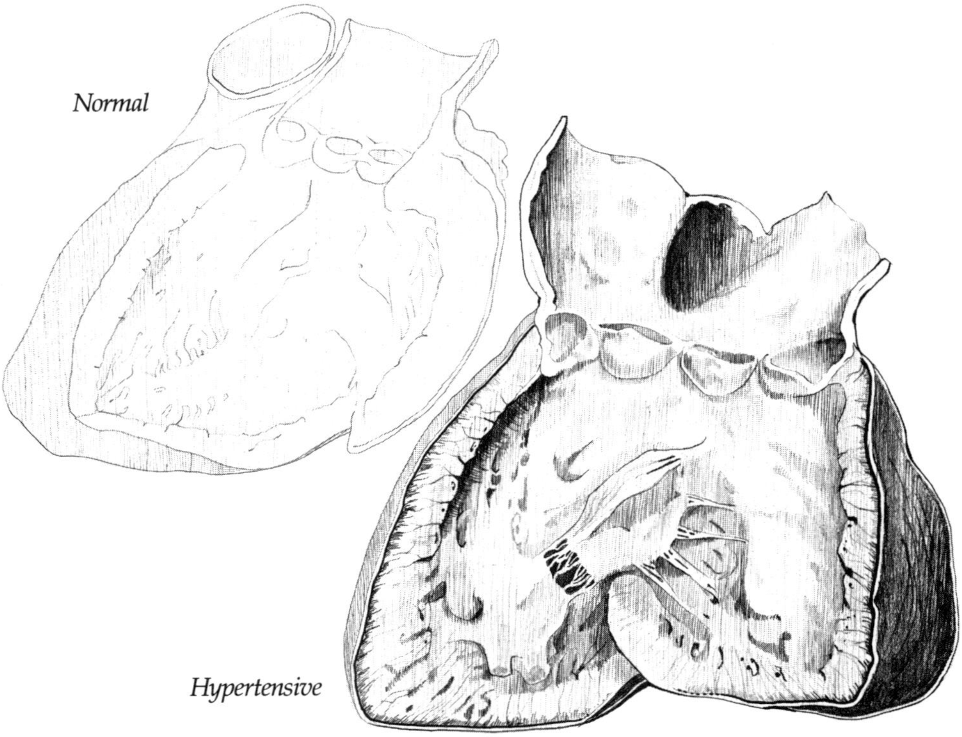

Because of the high pressure that it must pump against, the hypertensive heart becomes dilated and the muscular wall grows thicker.

Congestive Heart Failure

When people have hypertension, their hearts must work harder to pump the blood through the arteries. Over time, the heart enlarges to perform this task, but eventually there comes a point at which the muscle fibers of the heart stretch too far and the heart's pumping action becomes ineffectual. When the heart can no longer contract effectively, blood backs up into the lungs and the patient develops a cough and shortness of breath with the mildest exercise.

Because of the heart's inadequate pumping action, pressure builds up in the veins and capillaries of the body. When the pressure within the capillaries becomes elevated, an excess of water and dissolved salts is filtered through the thin capillary walls into the tissues. Under the influence of

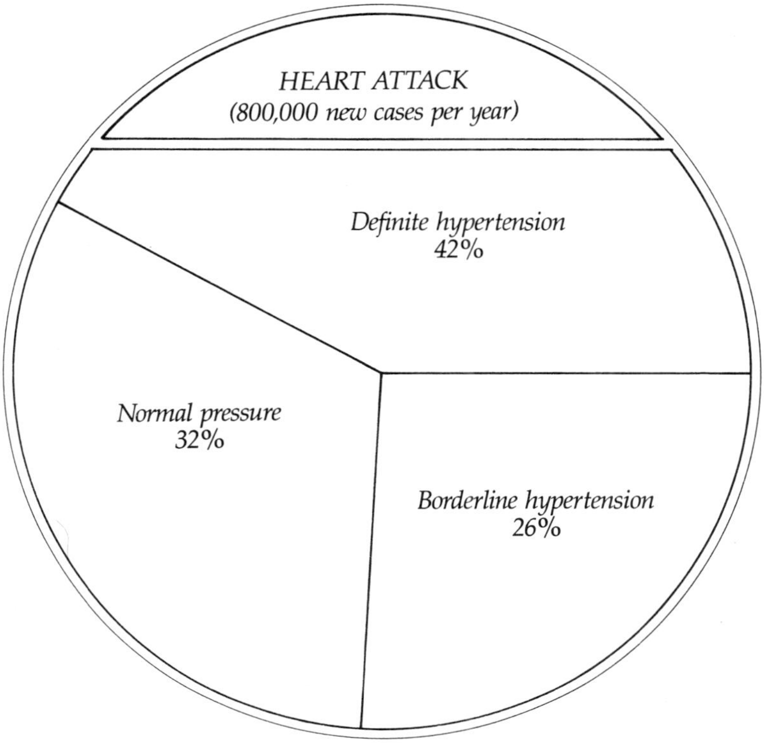

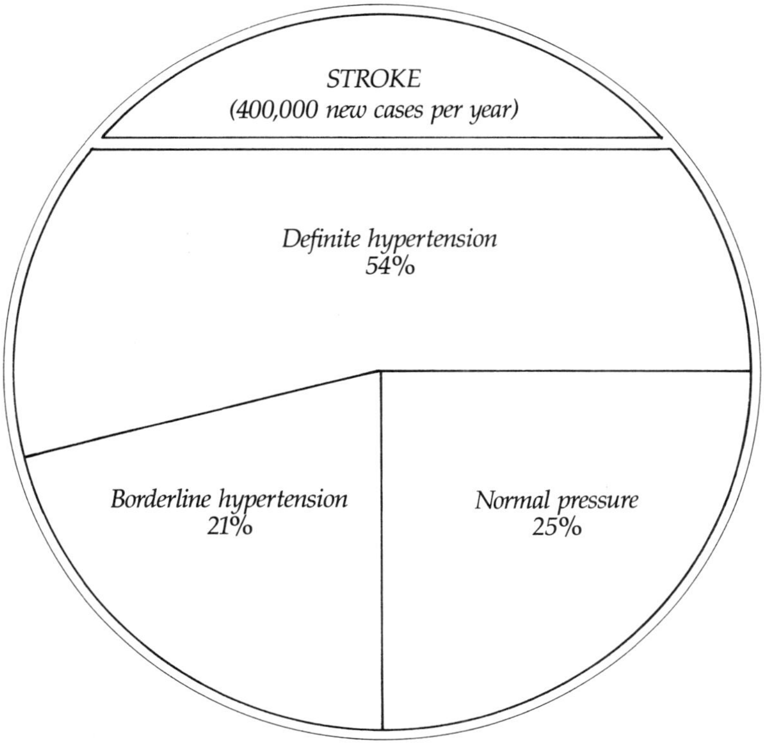

In the United States each year, 800,000 people have heart attacks for the first time. Sixty-eight percent of them have definite or borderline hypertension. Of the 400,000 people each year who have strokes for the first time, 75 percent have definite or borderline hypertension.

gravity, this excess fluid collects in the legs and ankles, causing swelling, or edema. In the advanced stages, the patient's complexion takes on a dusky, bluish tinge, called cyanosis, owing to the sluggish circulation of blood in the skin.

Congestive heart failure is a dire consequence of hypertension. According to William Kannel, the director of the Framingham study, *congestive heart failure is six times as common among patients with hypertension as it is among persons with normal blood pressure.* Once people develop congestive heart failure, they have a 50 percent chance of dying within the next five years, even if they are under medical care. Fortunately, treatment has improved in recent years and this disorder can be entirely prevented if the hypertension is controlled by medical treatment.

Strokes

Hypertension can damage the brain as well as the heart. It does so by causing strokes, which are due either to ruptures of brain arteries or to obstructions to them. This damage to brain arteries deprives parts of the brain of blood and the blood-deprived brain tissue dies.

Strokes are a serious health problem in this country. They are the third leading cause of death, following right after heart attacks and cancer. Those who survive a stroke may remain severely disabled, for once brain tissue has been damaged by a stroke, its function can seldom be completely restored.

Hypertension can cause strokes by so weakening brain arteries that they balloon out and burst, causing a hemorrhage that is usually fatal. Hypertensive patients also frequently develop microaneurysms (my-crow-an'-your-isms) of the arterioles. A microaneurysm is an outpouching of the wall of a brain arteriole, which may eventually burst, producing a hemorrhage.

Hypertension can also cause strokes by predisposing people to develop atherosclerosis in brain arteries. Atherosclerotic deposits narrow the arteries and may eventually block them. They are the cause of 57 percent of all strokes.

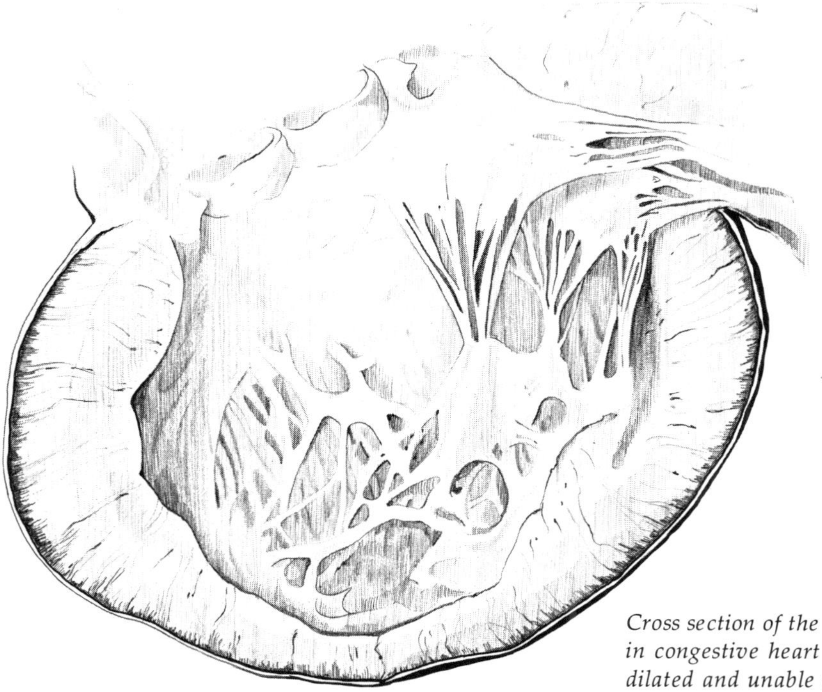

Cross section of the left ventricle of the heart in congestive heart failure. It is greatly dilated and unable to pump effectively.

The Framingham study showed that *people with hypertension are more than seven times as likely to have a stroke as are people with normal blood pressure.*

About 40 percent of the Framingham study participants who survived strokes required some sort of special nursing services for the rest of their lives. About 10 percent required total care for the rest of their lives.

Atherosclerosis and Heart Disease

People with high blood pressure are particularly likely to develop atherosclerosis, a disease in which the interior lining of the arteries is thickened by a fatty material called plaque. The thickening narrows the channel through which blood flows. Just as atherosclerotic plaques in the arteries of the

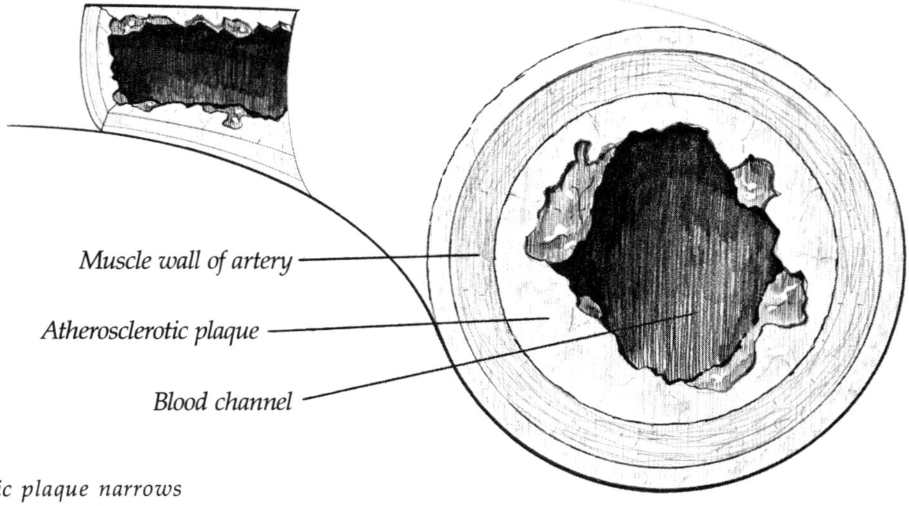

Atherosclerotic plaque narrows the channel through which blood flows in an artery.

brain can cause strokes, so can they cause heart attacks by blocking the blood flow through coronary arteries, which supply the heart muscle with blood.

There is no clear mechanism relating hypertension to the development of atherosclerosis. Medical investigators are not yet sure whether high blood pressure directly causes atherosclerosis or whether it indirectly predisposes people to develop atherosclerosis. The most popular theory today is that it causes atherosclerosis directly by injuring the inner lining of the arterial walls. Plaques then develop in response to this injury. This theory has not yet been proved, however, and it is not universally accepted in the medical community.

Whether a cause or a predisposing factor, high blood pressure is clearly related to atherosclerosis. There are three reasons for believing that this is so.

The first reason comes from animal studies. Animals in which high blood pressure is induced (by narrowing a kidney artery, for example) develop atherosclerosis. Animals with normal blood pressure that are reared under conditions similar to those of the hypertensive animals do not develop atherosclerosis.

Another reason to believe that high blood pressure leads to atherosclerosis has to do with the fact that the disorder normally does not develop in veins. The blood pressure in these vessels is always low, no matter what the pressure is elsewhere. Certain surgical procedures require the use of a vein to shunt blood past an obstruction in an artery. For example, in coronary bypass surgery, veins are grafted to coronary arteries to create passages through which the blood can flow. When the grafted veins are subjected to high blood pressures, they, too, often develop atherosclerotic plaques.

The third reason comes from statistical evidence linking hypertension to atherosclerosis. The Framingham study and similar investigations show that people with hypertension are more likely to develop atherosclerosis than are people with normal blood pressures, all other things being equal. The disorder is most likely to develop in coronary arteries of the heart muscle. In fact, in the Framingham study, the incidence of coronary artery disease, with resulting heart attacks, was higher than that of all other disorders linked to hypertension combined.

The Framingham results are dramatic. We have already seen how hypertension increases the risk of having a stroke caused by atherosclerosis. The increased risk of having a heart attack is equally impressive. According to the Framingham study, *men with hypertension are two and one-half times as likely to have a heart attack as are men with normal blood pressures. Women with hypertension are more than four times as likely to have a heart attack as are women with normal blood pressures*.

Kannel, as director of the study, was particularly impressed by the relationship of high blood pressure to atherosclerosis. He wrote, "Hypertension is powerfully related to the rate of clinical atherosclerotic events [strokes and heart attacks] and this relationship holds even when the impact of other major contributors is accounted for."

The likelihood that people with hypertension will develop atherosclerosis is increased even more if they have other risk factors as well. Among the best-established risk factors for atherosclerosis, in addition to hypertension, are heavy cigarette smoking, elevated cholesterol in the blood, and diabetes.

The more risk factors a person has, the more likely he is to develop atherosclerosis. For example, heart attacks before the age of sixty-five are rare in a person with no risk factors. But data from the Framingham study show that a forty-year-old man who has hypertension, who smokes cigarettes, who has diabetes, and who has a high concentration of cholesterol in his blood has a 60-percent chance of having a heart attack in the next eight years. On the other hand, a forty-year-old man whose only risk factor is hypertension has only a 3-percent chance of having a heart attack in the next eight years. If there are *no* risk factors present, the risk is less than 1 percent.

Other Complications of Hypertension

Heart attacks, congestive heart failure, and strokes are by far the most common effects of hypertension. But there can be other effects, especially if hypertension is not controlled.

One of these effects is kidney damage. The walls of the small arteries of the kidney become greatly thickened and the channels narrowed. The blood flow to kidney tissue is considerably reduced. As a result, the kidneys can no longer adequately rid the body of excess salt and water, and fluid begins to accumulate in the body. As conditions worsen, the kidneys may fail, resulting in uremic poisoning and possibly death.

Another effect of hypertension is eye damage. Fluid accumulation and hemorrhages from small blood vessels in the eye can obscure normal vision. This occurs only in the most severe form of high blood pressure, called malignant hypertension.

Very severe hypertension can also cause brain swelling due to fluid accumulating in the brain. A person with this condition, which is called hypertensive encephalopathy (en-seff-uh-lahp'-a-thee), may have a violent headache or convulsions or may go into a coma. Because of the extremely high blood pressure, a blood vessel in the brain may rupture, causing a cerebral hemorrhage, or there may be some other severe complication such as heart failure or kidney failure. Hypertensive encephalopathy is a medical emergency that requires immediate reduction of the blood pressure with antihypertensive drugs given intravenously. Fortunately, with early reduction of the blood pressure, patients will recover uneventfully.

CHAPTER 5

THE STORY OF DRUG TREATMENTS

A great medical achievement of our time has been the development of antihypertensive drugs. Just as the discovery of antibiotics ushered in a new era in the treatment of infectious diseases, so the discovery of antihypertensive drugs signalled a major advance in the treatment of cardiovascular diseases.

The years during which the antihypertensive drugs were developed were years of drama and suspense. With each new drug that was developed, doctors learned more about the disease of high blood pressure and more about how to forward the search for newer and better drugs. Although the drugs currently available are truly life-savers, the search for better drugs is not yet over. Drugs of the future promise to be even more effective and to have fewer side effects than do the current medications.

We would like to begin this chapter by telling you about the time preceding the development of antihypertensive drugs. The story of former president Franklin D. Roosevelt's losing struggle with high blood pressure illustrates the fate of many hypertensive patients at that time. It was shortly after this that medical investigators began to develop increasingly effective drugs to treat high blood pressure.

As one of the authors (Edward Freis) participated actively in the search for antihypertensive drugs from the beginning, we have written the story of how the drugs were discovered from his point of view, using the first person singular, so as to give you his personal recollections of this new era in medical history.

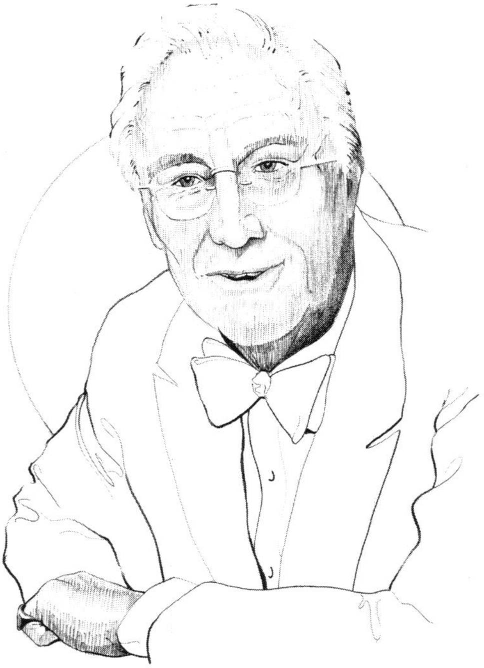

How Roosevelt Died

It was the spring of 1945, and President Franklin D. Roosevelt was not feeling well. His color was poor and he was very tired. His doctors prescribed a period of total rest; so he left Washington for Warm Springs, Georgia. For a few weeks after arriving in Warm Springs, the President seemed much improved. Then a catastrophe occurred.

On April 2, 1945, Roosevelt awoke with a slight headache. He attributed this to sore muscles, and felt better after he was massaged. He proceeded to go about his business, spending the morning going over State papers. As he worked, an artist sketched his portrait.

At 1:15 P.M., the president complained of a terrific headache centered at the back of his head. His physician, Howard G. Bruenn, recalls, "When I saw him, 15 minutes later, he was pale, cold, and sweating profusely. He was totally unconscious. . . . Systolic blood pressure was well over 300 mm Hg, diastolic was 190 mm Hg. It was apparent that the president had suffered a massive cerebral hemorrhage." Roosevelt never regained consciousness. At 3:35 P.M., Dr. Bruenn pronounced the president dead.

Roosevelt died of hypertension. Although his blood pressure was only 136/78 in 1935, it rose to 162/98 in 1937. Then it steadily increased, rising to an average of about 200/100 in 1944. Just before his death in 1945, Roosevelt's blood pressure varied markedly throughout each day. It ranged from a low of about 170/88 to a high of about 240/130. His doctors found no apparent cause for these blood pressure variations.

Bruenn served as Roosevelt's attending physician in the years preceding the president's death. Fifteen years later, he reported the history of Roosevelt's hypertension, writing, "As a result of this unforgettable experience, and as a practicing physician, I have often wondered what turns the subsequent course of history might have taken if the modern methods for the control of hypertension had been available."

Treatments "With a Pill and a Prayer"

The first effective treatments of hypertension were developed after World War II—a few years too late to help Roosevelt. Before that time, the diagnosis of severe hypertension was often a death knell. When patients had severe hypertension, physicians tried their best to keep the patients' minds off their blood pressures, fearing that, if patients kept track of their blood pressures, they might develop "manometer neurosis": that is, they might worry so much about their blood pressure that worry alone might cause their hypertension to worsen.

The conventional treatment for hypertension was with "a pill and a prayer." The pill was a mild sedative, such as phenobarbital, prescribed to keep the patient calm. Physicians also verbally reassured their patients and sometimes recommended that their patients see psychotherapists.

When hypertension progressed to a point at which a patient's organs were damaged and his life endangered, a physician sometimes resorted to more drastic measures. The patient was referred to a surgeon, who cut the nerves of the patient's sympathetic nervous system (a procedure known as sympathectomy). The patient was then put on a diet severely restricted in sodium.

Sympathectomy was truly a debilitating operation. The surgery itself was major and serious, causing severe blood loss. After the operation, the veins no longer constricted when patients stood up. Blood collected in their feet and legs, and they often fainted. To prevent fainting, many patients had to wear long elastic stockings and tight girdles. Some male patients could not ejaculate as a result of the operation. Patients also had trouble with control of their body temperatures, leading them to suffer chills in cold environments. In addition, patients had chronic pain along their ribs where the nerves were cut.

Nonetheless, sympathectomy saved some peoples' lives. For example, a U.S. senator came to Massachusetts Memorial Hospital during World War II in order to have this operation. The senator had severe hypertension at the time. He did quite well following sympathectomy and led a productive life for years.

The First Drug Treatment

The story of the first effective drug treatment of hypertension begins during World War II. Physicians testing the antimalarial drug pentaquine found that high doses of the drug lowered the blood pressures of normal volunteers.

It was at that time that my participation in evaluating drug treatment of hypertension began. I was a resident physician at the Massachusetts Memorial Hospital, working with physicians there and at the Squibb Institute for Medical Research. We wanted to explore the possibility of using drugs to treat high blood pressure. James Shannon, who was the director of the Squibb Institute, and later became the distinguished director of the National Institutes of Health, suggested that we try treating hypertensive patients with pentaquine.

We soon found that high doses of pentaquine did indeed lower the blood pressures of hypertensive patients. However, the doses required to lower their blood pressures produced such serious side effects that we could not recommend pentaquine as an antihypertensive agent. The major problem was that it damaged the patients' sympathetic nervous systems.

During the time that we were studying pentaquine, something happened that encouraged us to continue our search for better antihypertensive drugs. It began when a patient was referred to us for treatment of the most severe form of hypertension—that is, malignant hypertension. He was a physician who had come to the Massachusetts Memorial Hospital from California in the desperate hope that a sympathectomy might arrest the progress of his disease. But the patient's kidneys were already so badly damaged from his high blood pressure that we felt that he could not survive sympathectomy. We decided to give him pentaquine instead.

The pentaquine treatment produced remarkable results. The patient's diastolic blood pressure fell from 160 to 100 mm Hg. And, most important, his symptoms of malignant hypertension were relieved. His headaches got better, he no longer had blood in his urine, the hemorrhages disappeared from his eyes, and his congestive heart failure improved. This was the first time that we had seen a reversal of the signs of malignant hypertension following drug treatment. It was a most exciting experience and it convinced us that, if we could find drugs to lower blood pressure effectively and safely, we could prevent many of the complications of hypertension.

Unfortunately, our patient's kidney failure gradually worsened. He died several months later after returning to California. However, his final months of life were more comfortable than they would have been without pentaquine.

The Search for Drugs

Encouraged by our results with pentaquine, we began an intensive search for antihypertensive drugs. Working with another physician, Joseph Stanton, I combed the medical literature, hoping to come up with a useful lead.

We soon discovered reports of a drug called veratrum (vuh-ray'-truhm), which had been extracted from the herb *Veratrum viride,* that sounded promising. This drug lowered the blood pressure and had been used by nineteenth-century physicians to "soften the pulse" and lower the body temperatures of patients with fevers. Before that, *Veratrum* had been one of the medicinal herbs used by the American Indians.

We took up the study of veratrum and discovered that it was particularly helpful in patients with congestive heart failure. It not only lowered their blood pressure, but caused the signs of their congestive heart failure to disappear.

Our studies with veratrum led us to another exciting discovery. We found that, after lowering the blood pressures of some of our patients with drugs, we could do away with the drugs and their blood pressures would remain lower than they had been before.

We made this discovery when we treated a patient who had extremely high blood pressure. For some reason, this

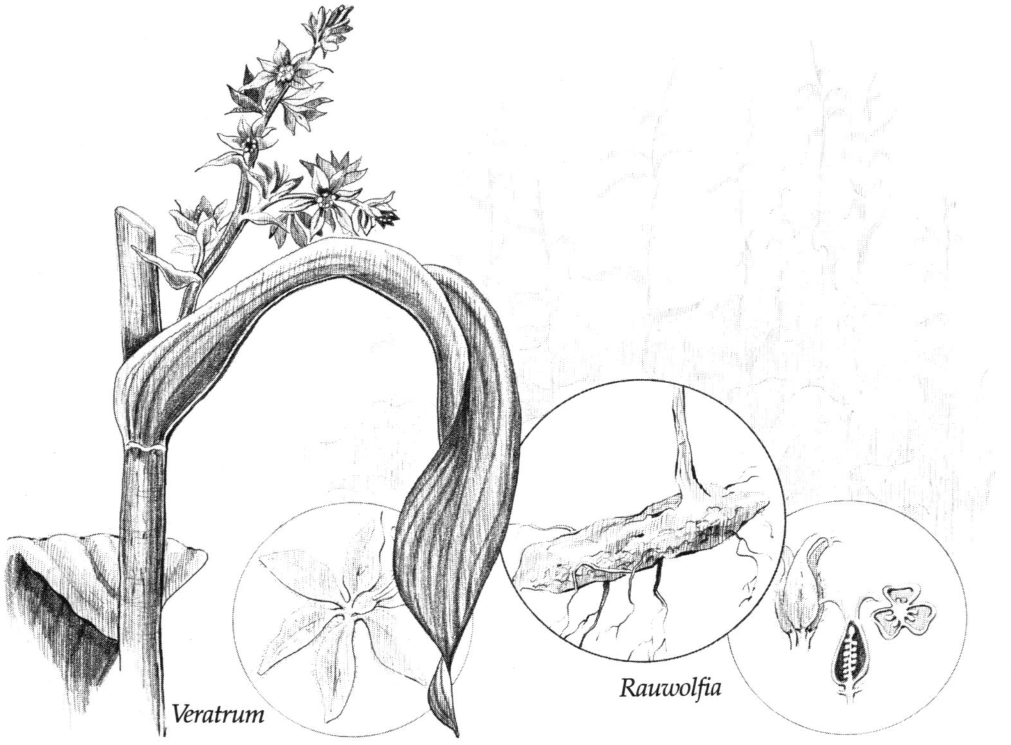

man stopped responding to oral doses of veratrum. However, he still responded to injections of the drug.

We began giving this patient daily injections of veratrum. Each day, his blood pressure fell after the injection and then gradually rose again. To our surprise, one week after we had begun the injections, the man's blood pressure reverted to a lower level rather than rising to severe levels between injections of the drug. He eventually left the hospital with his blood pressure fairly well controlled by a diet that was severely restricted in salt. Before the veratrum injections, the low-salt diet had not affected his blood pressure. (The patient was not able to do without treatment entirely, and from 80 to 90 percent of patients with moderate to severe hypertension cannot discontinue taking their drugs without risking serious consequences.)

Veratrum was no panacea, however. The margin between the dose required to lower blood pressure and the toxic dose was narrow and, in some cases, nonexistent. Patients would at times develop severe reactions including violent retching, sweating, salivation, abnormally slow heart rates, and low blood pressures. Finally, the patients would collapse. These attacks were short-lived, but they made the drug unacceptable for treating patients other than those with the most severe forms of hypertension.

Our next discovery was that a combination of treatments could be more effective than one treatment alone. We gave patients veratrum and a low-salt diet and found that their blood pressures were lower than when we gave them only veratrum. Then we combined treatments for patients whose hypertension seemed truly intransigent. These patients had failed to respond to low-salt diets, veratrum, or sympathectomy alone. However, their blood pressures dropped when we combined the three treatments.

As a result of these experiences, we were already searching for drugs that would chemically reproduce the effects of sympathectomy and low-salt diets. We tried a number of drugs, none of which seemed suitable for the long-term treatment of hypertension.

In 1950, two British investigators synthesized a new drug, hexamethonium (hex'-uh-meth-oh'-nee-um), that mimicked the effects of surgical sympathectomy. The drug seemed extremely promising because it decreased dangerously high blood pressures by blocking nerve impulses from the autonomic nervous system. But its side effects were so severe that it could be used only for the most seriously ill patients.

These side effects were vividly depicted by William D. Paton, one of the physicians who discovered hexamethonium, in his description of the "hexamethonium man."

> He is a pink-complexioned person, except when he has stood for a long time, when he may get pale and faint. . . . He may laugh, but he can't cry because the tears cannot come. . . . He dislikes speaking much, unless helped with something to moisten his dry mouth and throat. . . . He tends to get cold and keeps well wrapped up. . . . He is thin because his appetite is modest; he never feels hunger pains and his stomach never rumbles. He gets rather constipated, so that his intake of liquid paraffin [mineral oil] is high. As old age comes on, he will suffer from retention of urine and impotence. . . . One is uncertain how he will end, but perhaps if he is not careful, by eating less and less and getting colder and colder, he will sink into a symptomless hypoglycemic coma, and die, as was proposed for the universe, a sort of entropy death.

Although the description is somewhat exaggerated, it characterizes the difficulties that patients had with the side effects of drugs in the early days.

At about the same time as the discovery of hexamethonium, a far more promising drug, rauwolfia (rau-wool'-fee-ah), was discovered. Actually, the drug was rediscovered, for it was an ancient Indian sedative and remedy for insanity, hysteria, and epileptic fits. The drug itself is the powdered root of a shrub.

As early as 1931, two Indian physicians described the use of rauwolfia for the treatment of hypertension. But their report was published in an Indian medical journal and little attention was paid to it outside India. Then, in 1949, an Indian physician named Rustom Jal Vakil published another report of the use of rauwolfia in hypertension. This report was read by Robert Wilkins of Boston, who began using the drug to treat patients. He found that not only was rauwolfia effective, but it had fairly minor side effects when given in small doses. And its dosage could be decreased when it was given in combination with other drugs. The crude root is seldom used today, having been replaced by reserpine, which is the principal active ingredient.

Between 1952 and 1957, drug companies and medical investigators throughout the world intensified their search for antihypertensive drugs. The search was successful. Drugs were found that had tolerable side effects and that still blocked nerve impulses from the sympathetic nervous system. A very important group of drugs was discovered in 1958 that are known as thiazide diuretics (thigh'-uh-zide dye-your-ett'-iks); they mimic the effects of low-salt diets. Still other drugs were developed that act directly on the muscle coat of the small arteries to relax them. Drug combinations were discovered that allowed doctors to give small non-toxic doses of several drugs and still lower patients' blood pressures. For the first time, it was possible to control the blood pressures of a majority of patients with relatively little discomfort or inconvenience.

Within the brief span of five years, from 1952 to 1957, the drug treatment of hypertension had been revolutionized, allowing the use of a choice of drugs that were practical for the treatment of all forms of hypertension. True, some patients still had side effects from the new drugs. But they were far less common and much less severe than those we had seen before. Furthermore, the new drugs were more effective in controlling blood pressure. We were confident that the drug treatment of hypertension had truly come of age.

How Useful Are the Drugs?

The antihypertensive drugs were very effective in lowering patients' blood pressures. But the burning question of the decades between 1950 and 1970 was, Can the drugs prevent complications of hypertension and save lives?

Most physicians believed that the drugs prolonged the lives of a small group of patients—those with malignant hypertension. As noted earlier, this is a type of severe hypertension characterized by very high blood pressure, with eye changes, edema of the brain, and kidney failure. However, physicians were not sure that the drugs were equally useful in patients who had what is called benign hypertension—by far the most common form of high blood pressure. The name is unfortunate because it is certainly not a benign disease, given that it ultimately leads to congestive heart failure, heart attacks, and strokes. Unlike malignant hypertension, however it progresses slowly and it rarely causes death from kidney failure.

In 1963, I decided to determine how useful the drugs are in treating benign hypertension. The study was carried out in cooperation with medical associates who were in other Veterans Administration hospitals. We selected a total of 525 veterans, all of whom had benign hypertension. The men were randomly divided into two groups. Members of one group were treated with antihypertensive drugs. Members of the other group were given placebos (innocuous substances that do not have a medicinal effect).

Such a study is ethical only if physicians truly do not know whether the treatment is helpful. No physician can in good conscience deny patients a beneficial drug. But when we began our study, physicians had no way of knowing whether the antihypertensive drugs should be given to patients with benign hypertension. In fact, most of them believed that the major complications were not due to the elevated blood pressure. Drug treatment was often scornfully referred to as treating the blood-pressure machine, not the patient.

Soon after we began our study, we saw dramatic results in one subgroup of patients. These were the patients whose diastolic blood pressures before treatment ranged from 115 to 129 mm Hg. The protective effect of treatment was so impressive that we ended our study of patients in this subgroup after only twenty months. We could no longer justify giving any of these patients placebos rather than active drugs.

The rest of the patients in the study had diastolic blood pressures before treatment ranging from 90 to 114 mm Hg. Although the drugs were not as dramatically effective in these patients, they still considerably reduced the incidence of deaths and complications of hypertension. Nineteen patients in the placebo group died, but only eight in the treated group died. Projected over a five-year period, the results indicated that 56 percent of the untreated patients developed major complications of hypertension compared with only 18 percent of the treated patients, a ratio of three to one in favor of treatment. The most significant effects of the drugs were in those patients whose diastolic blood pressures at the start of the study were at least 105 mm Hg.

We concluded that the drugs were extremely effective in preventing strokes, congestive heart failure, and progressive kidney damage. We had no evidence, however, that the drugs prevented heart attacks. It may be that the patients in our study who experienced heart attacks already had atherosclerosis in their coronary arteries at the time the study began. The drug treatment may have begun too late to save them.

Drugs May Prevent Heart Attacks

In 1978, a group of Swedish physicians reported that antihypertensive drugs may prevent heart attacks. These physicians studied 1,026 hypertensive men living in the town of Göteborg, Sweden. They followed the men for more than four years. At the end of that time, 6.9 percent of the men in the control group had had heart attacks. In contrast, only 3.6 percent of the men in the group given antihypertensive drugs had had heart attacks.

The Swedish physicians pointed out that their results are different from those of the Veterans Administration study because the Veterans Administration study showed no effect of the antihypertensive drugs on heart attacks. They suggested two possible reasons for the different results. First, the Swedish men were given a different drug from that given the veterans. Second, the Swedish men had milder hypertension. Because hypertension in the Swedish group had not progressed as far as it had in the veterans, the physicians believed that the Swedish men may have been treated in time to arrest the progress of heart disease.

The Time Bomb

Even without the results of the Swedish study, those of the Veterans Administration study indicating protection against all major complications except heart attack are an impressive reason for treating hypertension. One person who was particularly impressed by the Veterans Administration results was Elliot L. Richardson, former Secretary of the Department of Health, Education, and Welfare. Richardson's father, a distinguished Boston surgeon, had been incapacitated by a stroke at a relatively young age and ultimately died as a result. Hence, it was no surprise that Richardson was well aware of the dangers of uncontrolled high blood pressure.

In 1972, shortly after the results of the Veterans Administration study had become known, Richardson addressed the National Medical Association at its annual meeting. He remarked,

> In the course of our efforts to bring better health to the American people, there comes a time when we are ready to turn knowledge effectively into practice. *Now* is such a time. *This* is the moment—which we must not let slip away from us—to go on the attack against the killer hypertension.
>
> To be sure, we have had no dramatic breakthrough as the development of a vaccine. Yet the knowledge we have accumulated about the disease and the treatment of it is nothing short of dramatic.

Richardson set up the National High Blood Pressure Education Program to inform physicians and the general public about the need to take hypertension seriously and to control it with medication. He concluded his speech by announcing this program with the following words:

> Looking at the problem another way, there are at least 23 million American adults walking around with a time bomb ticking away inside them—a bomb that can kill or cripple them at any time. Only half of them know about it, and only one in five is doing anything about it.
>
> As I see it, our job is to get to those other four out of five persons before the bomb goes off.

CHAPTER 6

WHAT DRUGS ARE AND HOW THEY WORK

John L., a middle-aged insurance salesman, looked and felt in the peak of health. Much to his surprise, when he had a routine physical examination, his physician told him that he had high blood pressure.

John's physician gave him a prescription for pills to lower his blood pressure and advised him to reduce his salt intake. But the pills made John feel worse rather than better. He felt tired and weak and began to suffer from headaches. In addition, his food seemed tasteless when he cut back on salt.

Rather than reporting the side effects of the pills to his doctor, John decided to stop taking the medicine and to resume salting his food. He felt fine for the next ten years, even though his high blood pressure was irreversibly damaging his body. Then he suffered a stroke that left him unable to use the right side of his body.

John is not solely to blame for his failure to take his pills and change his diet. His physician is also at fault. John was never told that, even though the pills may make him feel poorly for a while, they are necessary if he is to stay alive and avoid serious complications. His physician neither discussed the possible side effects of the drugs nor explained that, if John suffered from intolerable side effects, his prescription could be changed to other drugs that might be more acceptable.

Many physicians are now realizing that the patients who do best are those who know the most about their condition and the drugs used to treat it. Because it is so important to understand the antihypertensive drugs, we will describe them in some detail, including how they work. Then we will explain what you can do to help your physician treat you.

All drugs have two separate names: one is the generic name and the other is the trade, or brand, name. The generic name is the scientific name given to the drug at the time of its discovery. The trade name is given by the company that markets the drug. For example, hydrochlorothiazide (high'-dro-clor'-oh-thigh'-uh-zide) is the generic name of a popularly used diuretic. It is sold by several drug companies under different trade names, among them Hydrodiuril and Esidrix. In the following discussion, we will use the generic names only. Appendix D lists some of the trade names of common antihypertensive drugs.

How the Drugs Work

As explained in Chapter 1, blood pressure is affected by blood volume, by the activity of the sympathetic nervous system, and by the constriction and relaxation of the arterioles. Each drug used to treat hypertension acts on at least one of these three control systems.

The most important group of drugs is the diuretics. These drugs reduce the amount of salt and water in the body and thereby decrease blood pressure. The second group of drugs inhibits the activity of the sympathetic nervous system. The third group relaxes the smooth muscle cells ensheathing the arterioles (smallest arteries), thus causing the arterioles to increase in diameter and so lower blood pressure.

Physicians frequently combine drugs having different kinds of actions so as to get a more powerful antihypertensive effect. When drugs are combined, each drug can be given in a lower dose than if it were given alone. This is important because the lower the dose the fewer the side effects.

The standard way to treat high blood pressure is the so-called stepped-care method. The physician begins by giving the patient a diuretic. If the diuretic controls the patient's blood pressure, nothing more is needed. However, if the blood pressure is still too high, the physician adds a second-step drug, generally an inhibitor of the sympathetic nervous system. If the patient's blood pressure is not sufficiently lowered with these two drugs, a third-step drug is

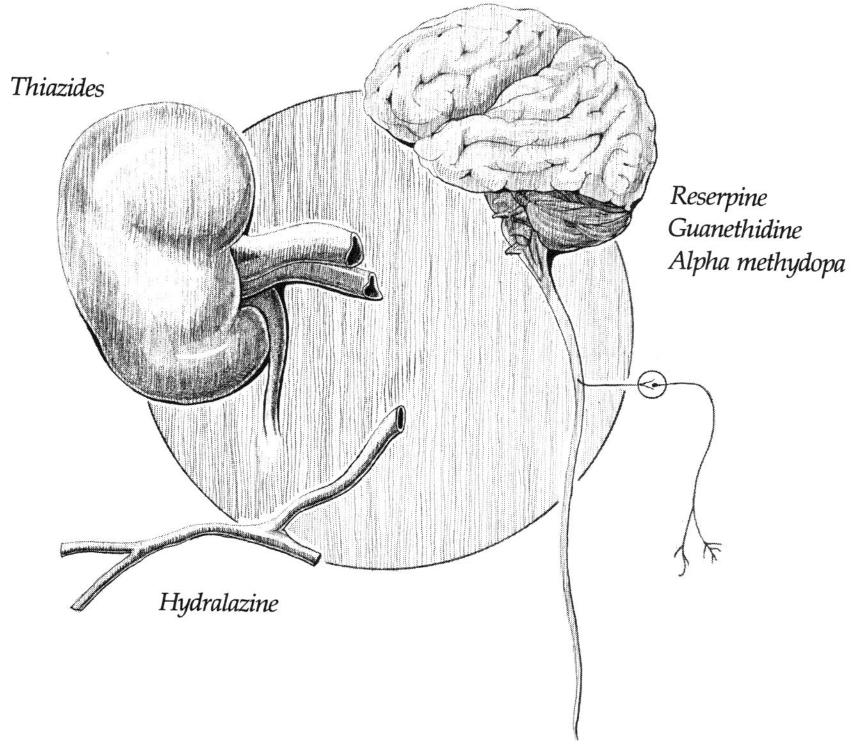

How the drugs act. Thiazides cause the kidney to excrete salt. Reserpine, guanethidine, and alpha methyldopa inhibit the sympathetic nervous system. Hydralazine relaxes the arterioles.

added, most often one that relaxes the smooth muscles encircling the arterioles.

Physicians almost always start the stepped-care program with a diuretic because these drugs have few side effects and because other drugs given alone often cause salt and fluid retention. Fluid retention can counteract the antihypertensive effects of the drugs, unless a diuretic is given at the same time.

The Diuretics

Many patients need take only a diuretic to control blood pressure. These drugs cause the body to excrete salt and water, producing an effect like that of a very low salt diet.

There are several kinds of diuretics, but those most often prescribed are the *thiazide diuretics.* These drugs are remarkably safe with few discomforting side effects. In the first two days of taking a thiazide diuretic, a patient may urinate a great deal. Then he probably will cease to notice any effects of the drugs.

The thiazide diuretics do cause patients to lose some potassium from their bodies, but this effect generally needs no treatment. Patients are sometimes told that they can prevent potassium from being lost by eating foods that are high in potassium. For example, they are told to drink a glass of orange juice or to eat a banana each day. Many doctors, however, believe that such dietary modifications are a gesture, not a treatment. You would have to drink at least ten glasses of orange juice or eat at least four bananas each day to obtain enough potassium to counteract the effect of the diuretic.

On the other hand, a low-salt diet does help prevent potassium loss. *More important, a low-salt diet increases the effectiveness of the diuretics, which can permit a reduction in dosage of the drugs.*

In general, the only patients who need to worry about potassium loss are those taking digitalis (dij-i-tahl'-iss), which is a drug used to treat congestive heart failure. When a patient is taking digitalis and loses potassium from his body, the digitalis can cause his heart to beat irregularly.

Patients who take digitalis *and* thiazide diuretics are often given a potassium supplement in the form of a potassium chloride solution. Another way that doctors treat such patients is to reduce their doses of thiazide diuretics and to add a second, mild diuretic of a type that prevents loss of potassium. These mild diuretics are referred to as potassium-sparing diuretics.

Some patients do not respond to thiazide diuretics, especially those whose kidneys are damaged. When this happens the patients are usually given other kinds of diuretics that act in a different way. For example, they may be given a *loop diuretic,* such as furosemide (few-roh'-suh-mide). Loop diuretics act on a part of the kidney known as the loop of Henle. They are extremely potent drugs—about twenty times as potent as the thiazides—and can therefore cause more serious side effects.

The Inhibitors

A number of different drugs inhibit the activity of the sympathetic nervous system. Some act on the brain centers, others act on the nerve endings. Still others block cells from responding to epinephrine and norepinephrine.

Brain Centers. One of the most widely used antihypertensive drugs is *methyldopa* (meth'-ill-doh'-pah), a drug that inhibits the brain centers controlling the sympathetic nervous system. Its most common side effects are sleepiness (this generally becomes less of a problem after about one week of therapy) and a dry mouth.

A drug similar in action to methyldopa is *clonidine* (klah'-ni-deen). It, too, commonly produces sleepiness and a dry mouth as side effects. Patients who must stop taking this drug are advised by their physicians to withdraw from it in gradually decreasing doses. Abrupt withdrawal may result in a sudden increase in blood pressure to very high levels.

Nerve Endings. Normally, the sympathetic nerves constrict blood vessels by releasing norepinephrine from their nerve endings into the wall of the blood vessel. Drugs that act on the nerve endings prevent norepinephrine from causing an increase in blood pressure. Some drugs do this by taking up the space on the nerve endings usually occupied by norepinephrine or by blocking the release of norepinephrine from nerve endings. Others deplete the nerve endings of their stores of epinephrine and norepinephrine.

The best-known but infrequently prescribed drug that blocks sites on nerve endings is *guanethidine* (gwah-neth'-i-deen). This is a very powerful drug that is generally given only to patients with severe hypertension. Its side effects include diarrhea and backward ejaculation in males (ejaculation is into the urinary bladder and so there is no emission). It can also cause patients to feel dizzy and faint when they stand up after arising from a prone position. One can see why this drug is reserved for the treatment of only the most severe cases of hypertension.

A popular drug that depletes nerve endings of their stores of epinephrine and norepinephrine is *reserpine* (reh-surp'-een). This drug is derived from the root of the plant rauwolfia.

The most common side effects of reserpine are nasal congestion, sedation, lethargy, weakness, and increased appetite with moderate weight gain. The claim that reserpine can cause breast cancer has not been substantiated. In some patients, reserpine can precipitate depression that, if not promptly recognized, can last for several months after the drug is withdrawn. When a patient on reserpine experiences depressed feelings lasting more than a day or two, he should inform his physician immediately to determine whether the drug should be stopped before the depression becomes established.

Sympathetic Nerve Blockers. Some drugs inhibit the activity of the sympathetic nervous system by preventing cells from responding to the nerve hormones epinephrine and norepinephrine. These drugs include *propranolol* (pro-pran'-oh-lol) and *prazosin* (pray'-zoh-seen).

Propranolol was first introduced as an antihypertensive agent in the United States in 1976. It had previously been used in this country in the treatment of heart disease. Propranolol is a very selective drug in that it prevents stimulation of the heart by sympathetic nerves but does not affect the nerves to the blood vessels. Thus, propranolol reduces the rate and the force of contraction of the heart. Another, similar drug is metropolol, and still others are being prepared for marketing.

Propranolol is contraindicated for patients with asthma, for patients with recent congestive heart failure, and for diabetic patients taking insulin. Its most frequent side effects are fatigue when exercising and cold hands and feet in extremely cold weather. It may also cause insomnia and nightmares.

Patients cannot suddenly stop taking propranolol without risking a heart attack. They must withdraw from the drug by taking gradually reduced doses for a period of several days or more.

Another drug that prevents cells from responding to epinephrine and norepinephrine is prazosin. However, prazosin acts on the blood vessels rather than the heart. First introduced in 1976, prazosin is frequently given to patients who cannot tolerate methyldopa or other inhibitors of the sympathetic nervous system.

Some patients taking this drug feel dizzy or faint when sitting up after lying down or standing after sitting. These reactions may disappear a few days after therapy is begun.

The Muscle Relaxers

The third class of drugs relaxes the smooth muscle cells surrounding the arterioles. As a result, the arterioles dilate, causing the blood pressure to fall.

The most commonly prescribed muscle relaxer is *hydralazine* (high-drahl'-uh-zeen). Its principle use is in combination with a diuretic with or without a sympathetic nerve blocker.

Hydralazine stimulates the heart through a reflex action on the sympathetic nervous system. The output of the heart increases and patients may sense this as a pounding or palpitation of the heart. These reflex effects on the heart are in large measure prevented if a drug that blocks the sympathetic nerves to the heart, such as propranolol, is given along with hydralazine. Hydralazine may also cause headaches, particularly in the first few days of treatment.

Hydralazine has an interesting history. It was popular twenty years ago but fell into disfavor when some patients had allergic reactions to it. Later these reactions were found to be preventable if smaller but still effective doses were

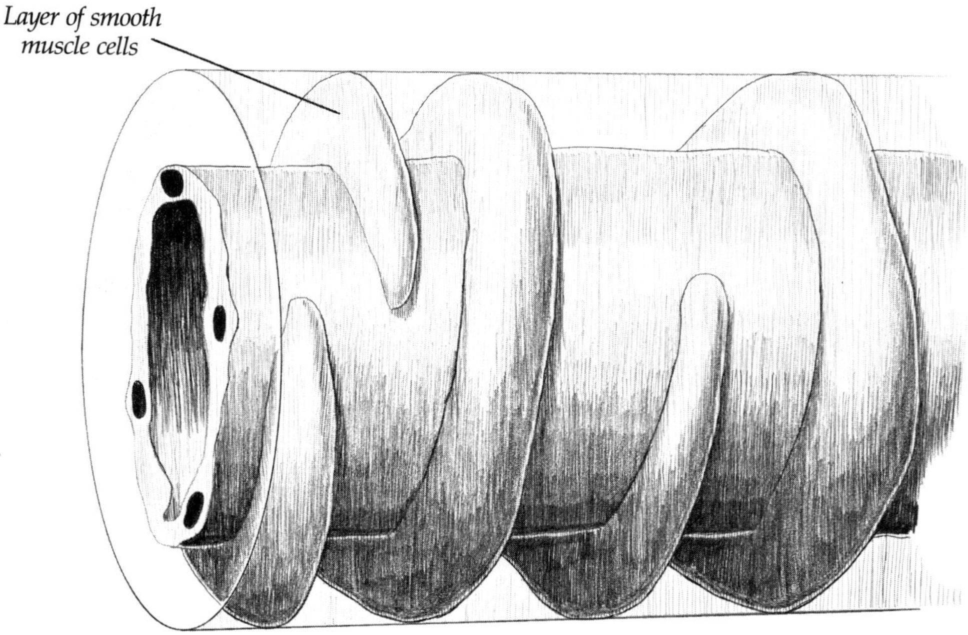

Section of an arteriole showing the smooth muscle that surrounds it.

used. Hydralazine, given in the smaller doses, again became popular about five years ago, when it was found that propranolol prevented the reflex stimulation of the heart.

New Drugs

Medical investigators are intensively searching for and testing new drugs for treating high blood pressure. A number of these drugs are available in Europe, although not yet in the United States.

Most new drugs for treating hypertension work along the same lines as the drugs now available. Their advantages are that they may have fewer side effects or may be effective in patients whose hypertension is not lowered by available drugs.

Recently, a promising new drug has been discovered that acts differently from all previously existing drugs. This drug, called *captopril* (cap'-toh-prill), seems to prevent the kidney hormone renin from causing blood pressure to rise. Its exact mechanism of action is not yet established, however. Scientists are hopeful that captropril will turn out to be more effective than other drugs currently in use.

How to Help Your Physician

You do not have to be a passive participant in programs to control your high blood pressure. There are a number of ways in which you can help your physician achieve that control.

If your physician prescribes a thiazide diuretic, you should cut down on salt. As mentioned earlier, low-salt diets increase the effectiveness of such drugs and often enable patients to get by with lower doses of them. And a low-salt diet reduces the possibility that you will lose an excessive amount of potassium when you take these drugs.

You may wonder whether you can drink alcoholic beverages when you take antihypertensive drugs. *In general, you can drink alcohol in moderation.* A few patients, however, feel faint when they drink alcohol while taking drugs that inhibit the sympathetic nervous system. If this happens to you, you should abstain from alcohol. The faintness is caused by the fact that alcohol itself causes blood vessels to dilate and thus lowers the blood pressure. The combination of the drugs and alcohol causes the blood pressures of some patients to drop too low.

Because patients with high blood pressure are susceptible to the development of atherosclerosis, you should make every effort to protect yourself from this disorder. *One of the most important things you can do is to stop smoking cigarettes.* Most medical scientists agree that people who stop smoking decrease their risk of developing atherosclerosis.

You may also want to follow a cholesterol-lowering diet, although these diets are somewhat controversial. There is no doubt that people with high concentrations of cholesterol in their blood are at high risk of developing atherosclerosis. The question is whether cholesterol-lowering diets will decrease that risk.

So far, there is no *direct* evidence that these diets will actually prevent atherosclerosis. Several studies have shown that a variety of cholesterol-lowering regimens, including diets, drugs, or a combination of the two, can reduce the amounts of cholesterol in the blood. But these reductions are usually modest—from 10 to 15 percent, for example. Some investigators consider these reductions to be so small as to make it impossible to demonstrate that cholesterol-lowering diets prevent atherosclerosis and heart disease.

Medical authorities who advocate cholesterol-lowering diets point out that the incidence of heart disease is lower in countries in which the national diet has little saturated fats and cholesterol. Moreover, diets high in saturated fats and cholesterol cause atherosclerosis in laboratory animals, including apes and monkeys. Jeremiah Stamler, a medical researcher at Northwestern University Medical School, says, "Long experience teaches that it is always dangerous to presume that man is completely exceptional and different from all other species, including other primates."

Cholesterol-lowering diets will probably do no harm, and so you may well decide to follow them. Many doctors agree with Irvine Page, a distinguished physician who is an expert in the cardiovascular field. He was for many years an active investigator of hypertension at the Cleveland Clinic. Page says he follows a cholesterol-lowering diet because he doesn't want to be the smartest man in the graveyard.

The most important way in which you can help your treatment is to *never change your medications without consulting with your physician.* You should not skip pills, because the timing of the doses of pills is designed to maintain the necessary amount of medicine in your body. If you skip pills, your blood pressure may rise, sometimes dangerously. You should not take it on yourself to stop taking your medication altogether. In some cases, such as when patients are taking propranolol, suddenly stopping the medication may even cause heart attacks. The medication is designed for a purpose and, if treatment is indicated, it will do you far more good than harm. The usefulness of the medication has been proved by carefully controlled studies showing that treatment protects against strokes, heart failure, and other serious complications of high blood pressure. But if you are remiss in your medication schedule, your blood pressure will not be well controlled and you will not be receiving the protection you deserve.

CHAPTER 7

WHAT GOES ON AT THE DOCTOR'S OFFICE

The attitudes of physicians toward the treatment of high blood pressure have changed dramatically in the past decade. As we have indicated, as recently as the late 1960s, many physicians felt that drugs for treating hypertension were of little, if any, value. Their whole emphasis was on identifying those rare patients who had curable forms of hypertension and sending them to surgery. A complete series of tests and examinations to detect curable forms of hypertension took from at least three to four days and was very expensive.

In 1970, the results of the Veterans Administration study of the treatment of hypertension were published. These results convinced most physicians that drugs for treating high blood pressure can save lives and prevent a great deal of suffering. Physicians no longer spend so much time looking for cases of curable hypertension. Instead, they generally use a few simple screening tests for these disorders, reserving the more complicated tests for young patients, who are more likely to have curable forms of hypertension, and for patients who do not respond to drug treatments.

In this chapter, we will describe what most physicians do in the course of examining a patient who may have hypertension. The first test is to be sure that the patient actually has hypertension. As will be seen later, not every person with one high blood pressure reading has hypertension. After being certain that sustained hypertension really is present, the physician ascertains the amount of damage that it has caused. Finally, he decides whether the patient should be treated and, if so, what treatment will be used.

Physicians differ in their ways of examining and diagnosing patients with high blood pressure. Because we cannot speak for all physicians, we will tell what one of the authors does when he examines hypertensive patients. As before, this chapter is written from Edward Freis's point of view, using the first person singular.

Do You Have High Blood Pressure?

Strange as it may seem, not all patients who are told that their blood pressure is high are actually suffering from hypertension. Let me give you an example. A woman was once referred to me by another physician. She was a school teacher in her early forties and was apparently healthy, but her case had driven the other physician to his wit's end. Whenever he measured her blood pressure, it was dangerously high. A typical value was 230/130. He treated her with every kind of drug but could not reduce her blood pressure.

When I examined the woman, despite the high reading, I could find no evidence that the high blood pressure had damaged her body. I became suspicious when the woman said she had a sister who also had high blood pressure and had been told by her physician twelve years earlier that she could not live six months with such an elevated blood pressure. She was, however, still alive and working. In fact, she had outlived the physician who had told her this.

It seemed likely that this patient, as well as her sister, was a hyper-responder; that is, a person whose blood pressure soars when it is being measured. At other times, when in a relaxed state, a hyper-responder has a much lower blood pressure or even a normal one.

I taught the woman how to take her blood pressure at home, where she would be more relaxed. After a few days, her blood pressure readings drifted downward. By the end of the second week, her blood pressure was normal and no treatment was necessary.

Because a number of patients are hyper-responders, I do not trust the results of one blood pressure measurement. I ask patients to return for as many as three visits. At each visit, I take the patient's blood pressure. If the pressure remains high, the patient probably has hypertension. But some patients are still apprehensive, even after three visits. When I doubt that a patient actually has hypertension, I teach the patient or, preferably, a member of his family to take his blood pressure at home, and then I instruct the patient to take a blood pressure reading in the morning and in the evening for two weeks. In most cases, if the patient is a hyper-responder, his blood pressure goes down to normal in this time.

There is some evidence that a hyper-responder is more likely to develop a sustained hypertension later on than are other people with normal blood pressure. Not all hyper-responders develop high blood pressure, but we want to find and treat those who do. I ask all hyper-responders to come back once a year so that, if they develop definite hypertension, I can detect it early. I even ask some hyper-responders to take their blood pressures at home several times each month and to report to me if their blood pressures go up.

How Much Risk?

If a patient has definite hypertension, the physician must decide whether to treat him and, if so, how. This decision depends in large part on how high the blood pressure is and how great the patient's risk is of suffering consequences of high blood pressure. The most important factor in determining risk is the level of blood pressure itself after several visits, mainly to eliminate the possibility that the patient is a hyper-responder. In general, the higher the blood pressure, the greater the risk.

But there are also a number of other risk factors. Other things being equal, the younger the patient, the greater the risk of the hypertension compared with normal persons in the same age group. Blacks are at higher risk than whites and males do not tolerate hypertension as well as females.

I also ask patients questions designed to help me assess other risks. For example, I ask whether the patient has a close relative who has had a complication of high blood pressure, such as heart disease, stroke, or kidney disease. If any of these complications has occurred in the immediate family, the patient's risk is increased.

Another important question is whether the patient has ever been told that he has high blood pressure and, if so, whether he has been treated for it. The longer his blood pressure has been high enough to warrant treatment and yet has not been treated, the more damage will have occurred to his heart, kidneys, and blood vessels and the greater his risk. If the patient has been treated, I want to know what the treatment was, when it was started, and how long it was continued. Most patients are treated with pills. If a patient was given pills, I want to know what they were, how frequently and consistently he took them, and whether they produced side effects.

Patients who have diabetes or high cholesterol or who smoke in addition to having high blood pressure are at an increased risk of developing heart disease. Therefore, I ask questions about these conditions. And I test for the presence of diabetes and high cholesterol.

Target Organ Damage

High blood pressure damages the brain, the blood vessels in the eye, the arteries, the heart, and the kidney. Such damage is called *target organ damage.* If it occurs, the patient is at increased risk of dying or becoming disabled from his high blood pressure. This is the kind of silent, slowly progressing damage that often leads to a major complication. I look for evidence of target organ damage and ask patients questions designed to find out whether such damage has occurred.

The Brain. Many people believe that if high blood pressure damages blood vessels in their brains they will have headaches. Actually, headaches directly related to hypertension occur almost exclusively in malignant hypertension. These headaches are of a specific type; they occur when the patients awaken in the morning and are located in the back of the head and neck.

When hypertension affects the blood vessels in the brain of a middle-aged or older person, his memory may fail him and his intelligence may be dulled. This is because of small strokes resulting from blocked or damaged blood vessels in the brain. Such patients act older than their age, have an unsteady gait, and may have a tremor.

I look for these signs of brain damage in my patients and I also ask if they have ever had a stroke, weakness, paralysis of any limb, or a blackout spell. These complications are also indications of brain damage caused by hypertension.

The Eyes. Frequently, the first signs of damage from high blood pressure are seen in the blood vessels of the eye. I shine a light into a patient's eyes and look at the arteriorles of the inner lining, or retina. If the arterioles are damaged by high blood pressure, their walls become thicker and harder. They then reflect more light than normal and indent the veins at points of crossing. When the blood pressure is extremely high for quite some time, as in malignant hypertension, small hemorrhages and whitish "exudates" may develop because of the damaged arterioles.

The Arteries. High blood pressure aggravates atherosclerosis, or hardening of the arteries. Therefore, atherosclerosis of the arteries of the neck, legs, and extremities is more common in patients with hypertension than in people with normal blood pressure. Atherosclerosis can cause narrowing or even blockage of these blood vessels. This causes the blood flow through the artery to become sluggish and the arterial pulse to be weak or absent.

To check for damage to the arteries of the legs, I feel the pulses in the feet and legs. If these pulses are not easy to feel, I suspect that there may be damage. I then ask the patient if he has pain in his calves when he walks, which can be a sign of poor circulation.

Patients with damaged arteries in their legs and feet are quite susceptible to infections of the toes and heels. I tell patients with atherosclerosis of their leg arteries to wash and dry their feet carefully and to avoid injuring or bruising their toes and heels. This is especially important in patients who are diabetics, because diabetes itself often damages the blood vessels in the feet.

I check a patient's carotid arteries in the neck by feeling the pulses in the artery on either side of the neck. If the pulse in the carotid artery on one side is weak and that in the carotid artery on the other side strong, one of these arteries may have undergone significant damage. I also place my stethoscope over each carotid artery. If the carotid artery has been severely narrowed by atherosclerosis, I can hear a murmur as the blood jets through the narrowed segment.

The Heart. In Chapter 4, we told you about the two kinds of heart disease that may be found in patients with untreated hypertension. These two conditions are congestive heart

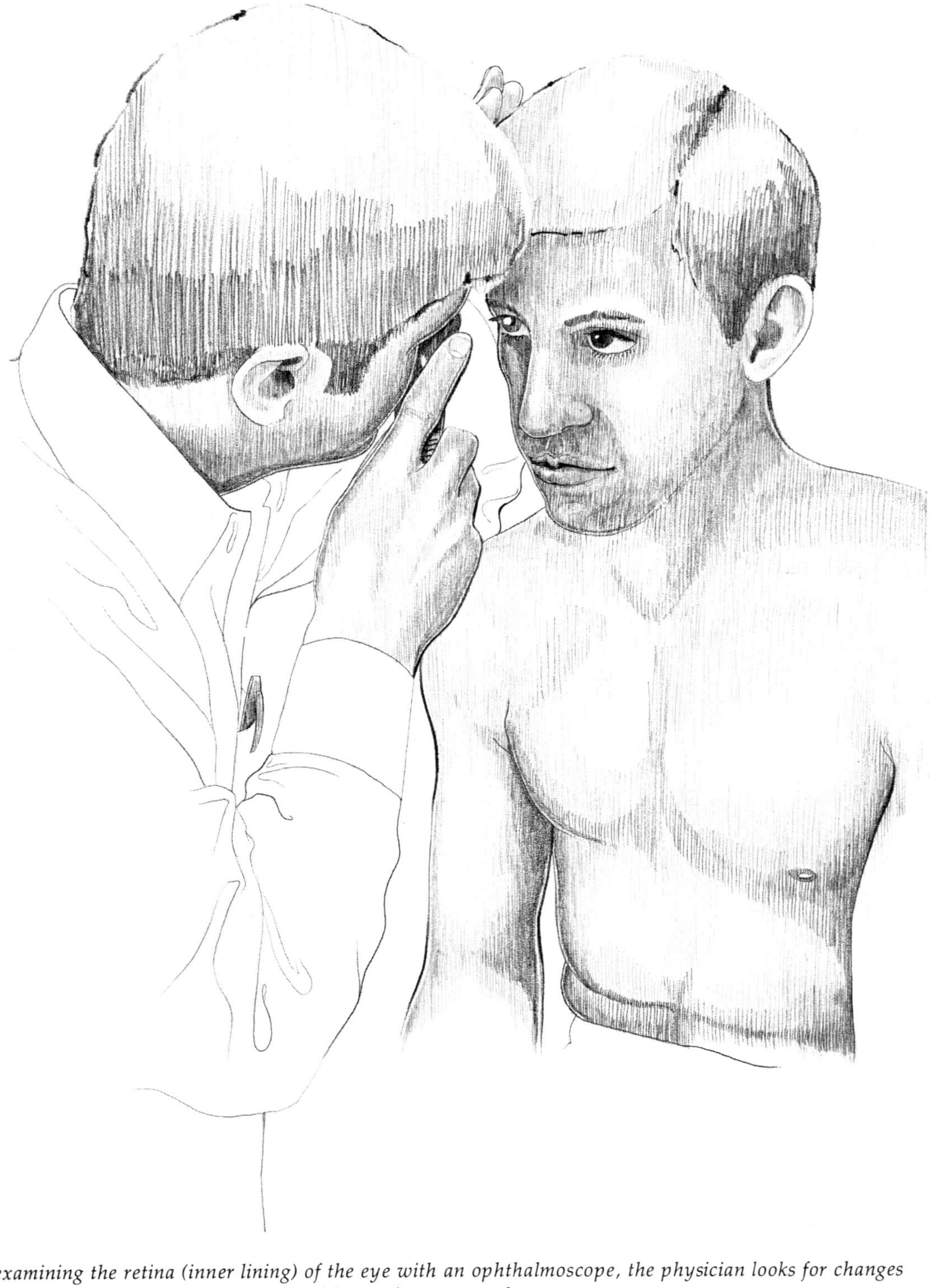

In examining the retina (inner lining) of the eye with an ophthalmoscope, the physician looks for changes in the arterioles and for the presence of hemorrhage or exudates.

failure and atherosclerotic heart disease (angina or heart attacks). The two case histories that follow illustrate the different symptoms of these two forms of heart disease.

The first case history describes a patient of mine who developed congestive heart failure. Russell M., a fifty-two-year-old building contractor, was a very busy man, too busy in fact to have a medical check-up. He had hypertension but did not know it. The first symptom that he noted was one that is commonly indicative of the onset of congestive heart failure. What he experienced at that time was a gradually decreasing tolerance of exercise, which was indicated by shortness of breath on less and less demanding exercise. He attributed this change to being overweight and to smoking cigarettes. But his shortness of breath became worse. Then he noticed that his ankles and feet became swollen during the day so that it was difficult for him to take his shoes off at night. He also became short of breath when he lay flat in bed and he had to prop himself up with several pillows. Alarmed by these symptoms, he finally came to see me. I found that he had severe hypertension, which had caused him to develop congestive heart failure. Russell is much more careful now about obtaining regular medical care.

The next case history is that of Rhoda T. Her symptoms typify those of the other major heart complication, atherosclerotic heart disease. This condition narrows the coronary arteries that feed the heart muscle. Although it can occur in patients who have normal blood pressure, it is much more common in those who have high blood pressure. Rhoda T. was forty-six years old. She was first told that she had hypertension ten years earlier, but she did not like taking drugs for it and she went for long periods without treatment. She felt well during this time until one day while running for a bus she noticed a constricting heavy sensation under her breastbone that forced her to stop and walk slowly the rest of the way. Attacks like that one became more frequent and were brought on with increasingly less exertion. Sometimes she would feel pain not only in the chest, but also running down the inside of her left arm. When she had these attacks, she would stop and rest and they would go away within a few minutes.

One evening, while watching television after a heavy meal, she experienced a crushing chest pain that was much more severe than any she had undergone before. At the same time she felt weak and short of breath and she broke out into a cold sweat. This time the pain did not pass but persisted for more than one hour. She was rushed to a hospital where tests indicated that she had had a heart attack.

Rhoda's first chest pains, occurring with exercise and relieved by rest, were due to an insufficient flow of blood through the narrowed coronary arteries, which were unable to meet the increased demands on the heart muscle caused by exercise. This condition is called angina. The more severe chest pain, which persisted despite rest and which was accompanied by other disturbing symptoms, indicated that, because of the severe narrowing of a coronary artery and the consequent stoppage of blood flow, a part of the heart muscle was receiving virtually no blood. Without a blood supply, that part of the muscle died. In such cases, if the dead area is small, the patient will usually make an uneventful recovery but, if it is large, the patient will often be seriously disabled thereafter or may even die during the attack.

When I examine a patient I look for signs of both of these very different forms of heart disease. The history is most important because of the great difference in symptoms of each of these two heart conditions. Patients with congestive heart failure will also have enlarged hearts, which show up on the x-ray of the chest or in the electrocardiogram. The symptoms of angina or of heart attack related to atherosclerotic heart disease are the most important part of the examination. In addition, the electrocardiogram will often yield evidence of deficient blood flow to the heart muscle or of an old heart attack.

The Kidneys. In Chapter 3, we described how certain disorders of the kidney, such as glomerulonephritis or narrowing of the artery to the kidney, may result in hypertension. The reverse is also true. Hypertension in and of itself may effect changes in the small arteries of the kidney that will damage the kidney to the point at which it can no longer function normally. This effect on the kidneys is usually seen in patients with severe hypertension.

To find out if there is an underlying kidney disease, I ask the patient whether he has ever been told that he had kidney disease, or whether he has had blood in his urine, a burning sensation when he urinates, kidney stones, a kidney infection, or prostate trouble. I also ask whether he has to urinate often at night (this could be a sign of either heart failure or kidney failure), though it usually means nothing more than that the patient sleeps poorly.

Who Should Be Treated?

Until fairly recently, most doctors hesitated to treat older people who had hypertension. Norman Kaplan, at the University of Texas Southwestern Medical School, has commented that, "As I grow older, I am more and more disturbed by the position that 'old people aren't bothered by their hypertension, and, besides, they have to die of something.' (That's an almost literal quote from a standard text on hypertension.)"

Now most doctors believe that anyone—old or young—who has moderate or severe hypertension should be treated. That means anyone whose diastolic blood pressure is 105 or greater. It is in patients with borderline and mild hypertension whose diastolic blood pressure is between 90 and 105 that controversy over treatment exists.*

The controversy arises because there is no convincing evidence that treating all people with borderline hypertension will save their lives and prevent complications of high blood pressure. Some patients may be helped but others may suffer more from the side effects of the drugs than from borderline hypertension.

There is no doubt that patients with borderline hypertension are at greater risk than those with normal blood pressure. For example, the Framingham study showed that patients whose diastolic blood pressure was from 90 to 94 had a 50 percent greater chance of having a stroke than did patients with normal blood pressure. Those whose diastolic blood pressure was 100 to 104 had a 300 percent greater chance of having a stroke than did people with normal blood pressure. But no one knew whether treatment of borderline hypertensives would always reduce their risk. This is because the studies that had been done, although showing great benefit from treatment in definite hypertension, failed

* Just as this book was going to press, Ralph Reader, Director of the Management Committee of the Australian Blood Pressure Study, announced the results of a trial that included more than 100,000 patients with hypertension. After 3.8 years of follow-up, the investigators found that, among patients with diastolic blood pressures of 100 mm Hg or higher, protection against major complications was three times as great for those treated as for those who were not. It was only among patients with diastolic blood pressures less than 100 mm Hg that they could not detect clear evidence for a protective effect. In view of these results, all patients with blood pressures of 100 mm Hg or higher should be considered to need treatment.

to produce convincing evidence of benefit in borderline hypertension.

Recently, the National High Blood Pressure Education Program and the drug firm Ciba sponsored a conference on whether or not to treat patients with borderline hypertension. H. Mitchell Perry, Jr., of the Department of Medicine at Washington University in St. Louis introduced the conference. He said,

> The management of mild hypertension has become a major dilemma in modern medicine. Should there be a general recommendation *to treat* with antihypertensive drugs, recognizing the lack of knowledge that such treatment is beneficial and recognizing that it will almost certainly produce some unwanted effects? Should there be a general recommendation *not to treat,* realizing that this might be withholding significant benefits, possibly [risking] myocardial infarction [heart attack]? Or should we attempt to determine if treatment is beneficial before making any general recommendations; unfortunately, to obtain this information will be very expensive and require many years.

However, there are studies underway now that are specifically aimed at the question of whether borderline hypertension should be treated. These studies should give us the evidence that we need within a few years.

The Coordinating Committee of the National High Blood Pressure Education Program could not reach a consensus on when to treat patients with borderline or mild hypertension. It recommends that physicians should decide on treatment on the basis of the individual patient's needs. But they do not suggest any guidelines to help physicians decide whom they should treat.

I believe that there are in fact some useful guidelines that physicians can use at the present time to help decide which patients with borderline hypertension to treat. There are certain risk factors that, if present, indicate that patients with mild hypertension may be adversely affected if they are not treated. For example, men are at greater risk than women, being one and a half times more likely to die from high blood pressure than are women. Blacks are at greater

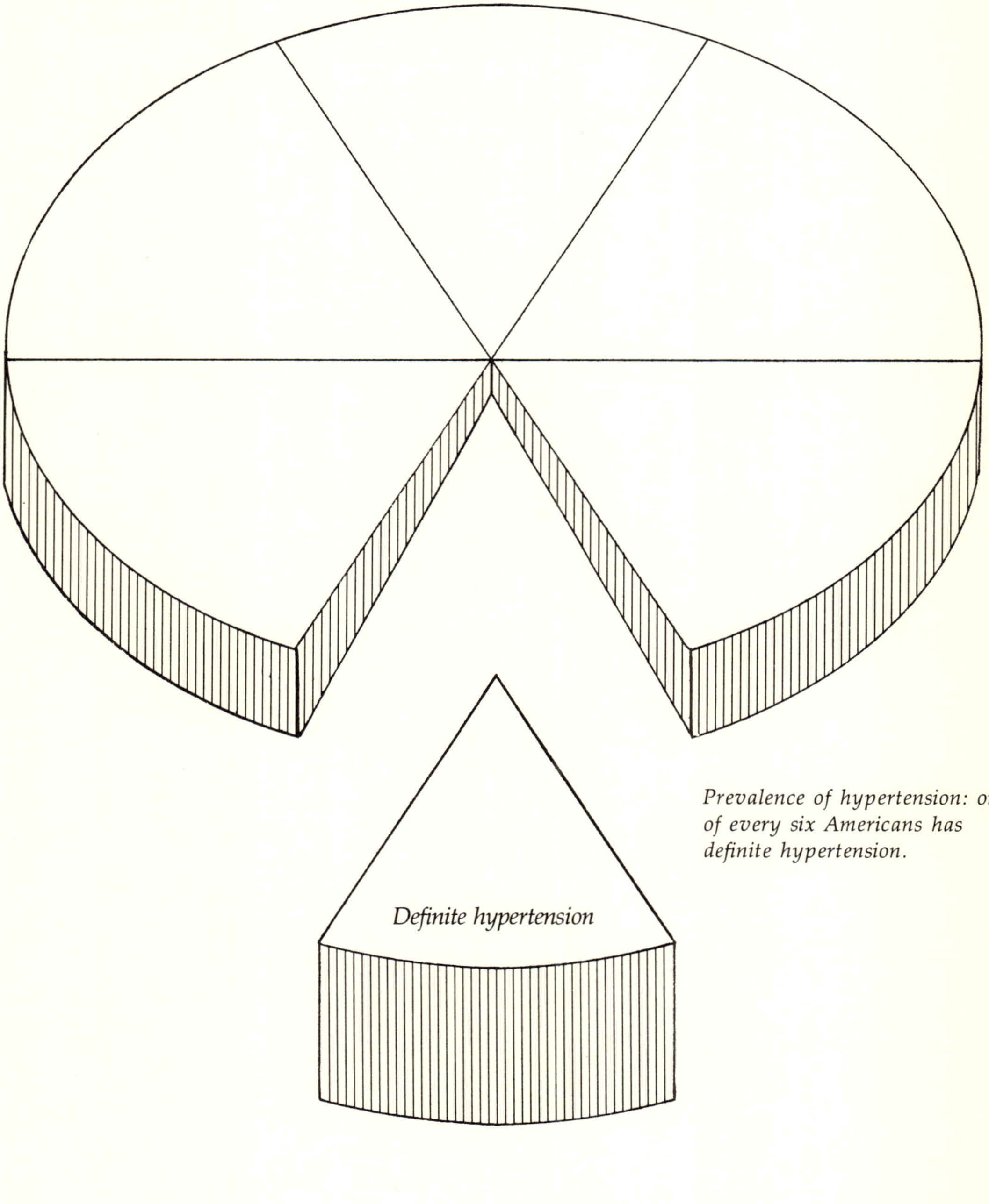

Prevalence of hypertension: one of every six Americans has definite hypertension.

risk than whites. Death rates from hypertension are more than twice as high among blacks as they are among whites. Age also confers risk, but it is the reverse of what you might think. The younger the patient, the more severe the consequences of hypertension. A man between the ages of thirty and thirty-nine with diastolic blood pressure of 95 is nearly three times as likely to die within the next twenty years as is a man of the same age whose blood pressure is normal.

Patients who have target organ damage (brain, heart, kidney) are at far greater risk than those who do not. Patients whose close relatives have had hypertension with serious complications are also at increased risk.

Physicians often weigh these risk factors when deciding whether to treat patients with mild hypertension. In patients with mild hypertension, the progression of their disorder is very slow. There is no urgent need to begin treatment immediately, and so the physician may wish to observe some patients for a time without treatment. He may see these patients every six months or every year in order to see whether their blood pressures are getting higher, staying the same, or drifting toward normal. But mild hypertensives who have several or many risk factors are apt to progress to a more severe hypertension.

I have devised a method to guide me in deciding which of my patients to treat. The scheme is based on risk factors that worsen the prognosis for hypertension. First, I measure the patient's blood pressure for at least three separate office visits. Those whose diastolic blood pressures average 100 or greater are treated, regardless of their other risk factors. Those whose diastolic blood pressures average less than 90 are not treated, regardless of other risk factors.

For the patients whose blood pressures average between 90 and 100, I use a scoring system to help me make a decision. I assign the patients points for the presence of risk factors according to the following table:

Risk Factor	Points
Age: Less than 50	1
Race: Black	1
Sex: Male	1
Target organ damage	2
All diastolic blood pressure measurements above 95	1
Family history of hypertension	1

I add up the patient's points. If the sum is 4 or more and the patient's diastolic blood pressure is between 90 and 94, I advise treatment. If the score is 3 or more and diastolic blood pressure is from 95 to 99, I also advise treatment. If the score is 2 or more and diastolic blood pressure is 100 to 105, I will treat the patient.

Other physicians, of course, have other ways of deciding whom to treat. My method is not the only way and, in fact, is a bit more conservative than others. Because the whole question of treatment for mild or borderline hypertensives is so controversial at the present time, you need not expect your physician to follow these guidelines.

Treatment

I generally give a patient a thiazide diuretic to start with. If this does not control his blood pressure, I add other drugs, as discussed in Chapter 6.

It is very important that a patient understands what blood pressure is, why high blood pressure is a serious condition, and how the treatment will help. Therefore, I spend some time explaining these things to the patient. I emphasize that, if his blood pressure is reduced to normal, he should expect to live out a normal life span in sound and vigorous good health. I also explain the most severe side effects of the patient's medication and ask him to contact me immediately if any of those side effects occur.

I always rely on a nurse to help me educate my patients about high blood pressure and its treatment. The nurse also checks the patients' blood pressures and quizzes the patients on the types of drugs they are taking and the presence of side effects. Nurses are very important providers of medical care in the long-term management of hypertension. In fact, there is evidence that nurses do a more thorough job of *routine* care and follow-up than do physicians. Once the nurse and I have examined the patient and explained why and how he is to be treated, we send the patient home, with instructions to return at regular intervals for check-ups.

Patients who understand why they are being treated and who cooperate with the treatment programs designed for them do very well. For example, one of my patients who is now seventy-six years old was referred to me in 1952 with severe hypertension and a blood pressure of 220/140. At first, we had no good drugs for treating him, and he had to inject himself twice a day with hexamethonium—a drug with debilitating effects.

Now this patient takes pills with fewer side effects than hexamethonium. He takes his pills religiously and he takes his own blood pressure at home to make sure it stays under control. Not only is he alive and well, but his blood pressure remains normal. He is the chairman of the board of a major hotel and goes to work every day, continuing to lead a fruitful and productive life. Without treatment, he could not have lived more than a year or two with such severe hypertension as he had in 1952.

CHAPTER 8

CHANGES IN LIFE-STYLE

Drugs have revolutionized the treatment of high blood pressure, but drugs alone are not the complete answer to the treatment of the disease. *There are a number of changes in life-style that can, in some cases, reduce the amount of drugs needed for the control of high blood pressure. In addition, these changes could conceivably help prevent high blood pressure if undertaken early in the natural course of the disease.*

In this chapter, we will tell you why certain changes in life-style may be helpful and how you may accomplish them. We will also describe changes in life-style that have *not* been shown to be helpful, although they have been advocated for hypertensive patients.

Some of the changes we will suggest may sound difficult to accomplish. Many people, in fact, hesitate to even think of changing habits of a lifetime, fearing that they will never succeed. This fear is not unreasonable for it is unfortunately true that not many who say that they want to change their habits actually do so.

Yet we know that some people are able to permanently change their habits. What distinguishes them from the many others who fail to break lifelong habits? Studies indicate that those who succeed are the ones most committed and most determined to change. According to Gloria Leon, a psychologist at the University of Minnesota, people who succeed in changing lifelong habits make a *firm personal decision* to change. Once this decision is made, success is almost assured.

Eating Less and Exercising More

Of all the changes in life-style that have been suggested, those that result in a loss of weight are the most important. There is good evidence that excess weight itself leads to high blood pressure. Not only are overweight people more prone to develop high blood pressure, but those who lose weight stand a good chance of lowering their blood pressures.

Leading specialists in hypertension believe that weight loss is the most effective way to lower blood pressure short of taking drugs. In fact, the Israeli study discussed in Chapter 2 showed that some patients who lost weight lowered their blood pressures so much that they no longer needed to take drugs!

Many people, however, fervently want to lose weight but are not able to do so. Every time they lose weight, they soon regain it. Often these people try one quick-weight-loss scheme after another, not realizing that such schemes are not only useless in the long run but may be dangerous as well.

One particularly harmful quick-weight-loss scheme is to take amphetamines, better known as "diet pills." *People who take these pills are no more likely to lose weight and maintain their reduced weight than are people who do not take them.* In fact, the Food and Drug Administration wants to ban the use of these drugs for dieters not only because they are ineffective, but also because they are addictive and have deleterious effects on the body. For example, they speed up the heart rate, which can be dangerous for anyone with heart disease. They are particularly harmful in hypertensive patients because they tend to raise blood pressure.

Less harmful, but also useless, are over-the-counter diet pills. These pills are generally made of indigestible fiber that expands in the stomach, making the dieter feel full. Unfortunately, however, studies have shown that people soon become accustomed to this feeling of fullness and resume eating as much as ever.

Drug stores also sell diet candies that are supposed to suppress the appetite. These are merely candies supplemented with vitamins and minerals. Needless to say, they have no effect on the appetite.

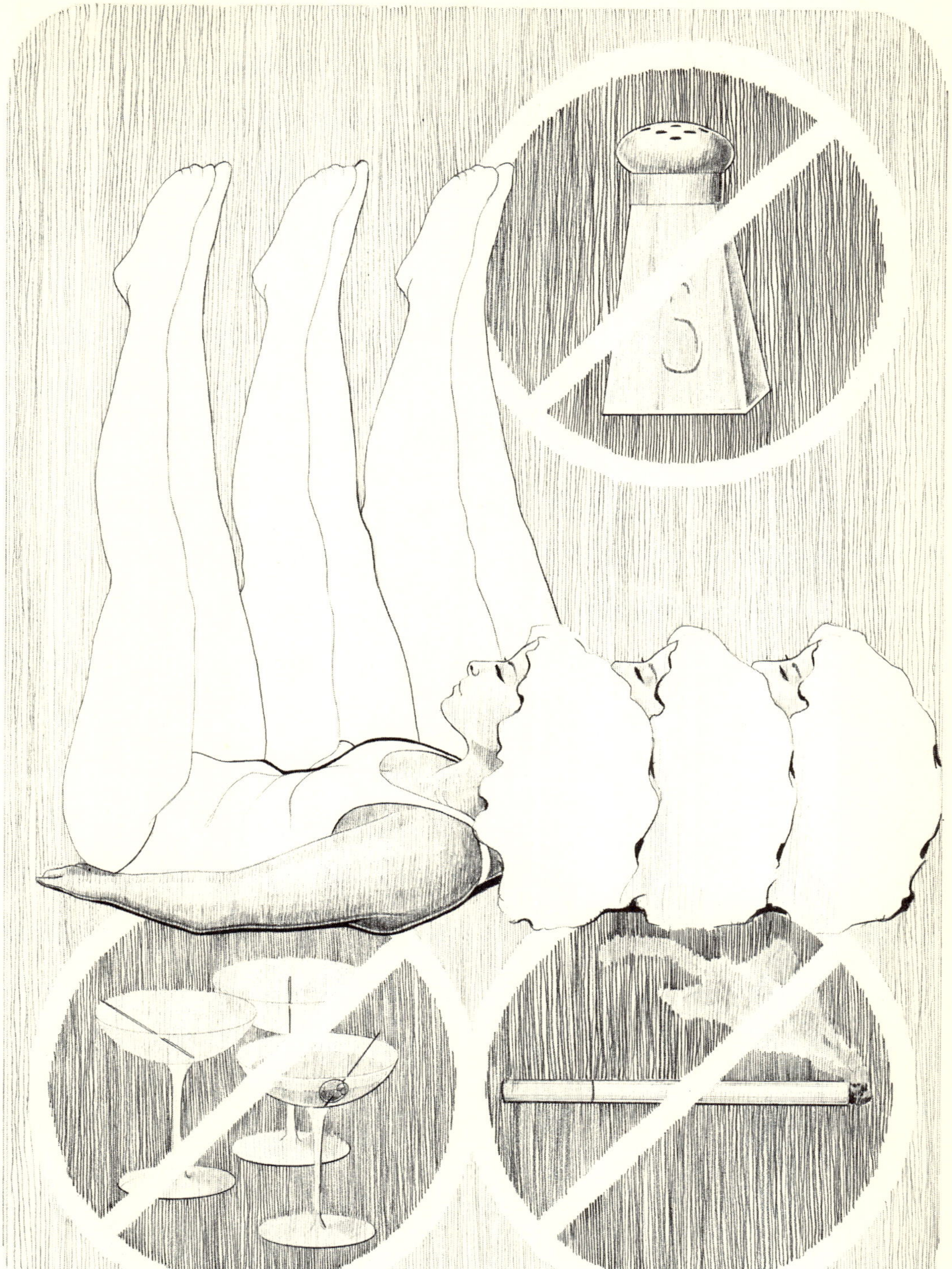

Preventive measures: maintaining a normal weight by eating less and exercising more; restricting salt consumption; limiting alcohol consumption to one or two drinks per day; and no smoking.

Other quick-weight-loss schemes are crash diets. Some of these diests, such as fasts and "liquid protein" diets, have been shown to be harmful. In fact, some patients on the liquid-protein diets have died, even though they were under the care of a physician. Other crash diets strictly limit the amount and variety of food to be consumed. These diets are difficult to follow for any length of time and can badly affect your health.

What is needed for lasting weight loss are permanent changes in eating habits and activity patterns. In other words, if you are overweight, don't think of "going on a diet" as a temporary period of deprivation. Instead, think of losing weight as a positive and permanent change in food choices that will make you feel better and look better, and will probably lower your blood pressure as well.

Many people find that they are able to change their eating habits permanently with the aid of the diets, behavior modification techniques, and group support of a commercial diet club, such as Weight Watchers, TOPS, or Diet Workshop. Club members learn about why they overeat and how to stop overeating. They also learn how to choose a nutritionally balanced diet that will enable them to lose weight. Having lost the weight, members are able to maintain their reduced weight by slightly modifying that diet.

Other people find that weight-loss clubs are not for them. They prefer to learn about nutritionally balanced diets on their own so that they can change their eating habits according to their own design. These people can obtain information on how to lose weight from the local chapter of their American Heart Association or from books available in their local libraries or bookstores promoting well-balanced (not fad) diets.

Whether you decide to lose weight with a group or on your own is unimportant. What is important is that you make a firm and lasting commitment to learn new eating habits.

You will greatly aid your weight-loss program if you also exercise regularly. Many people think that exercise only increases the appetite or that it takes so many hours of vigorous exercise to lose a pound that it is not worth the effort of trying. However, a little exercise every day burns up enough extra calories so that some weight will be lost gradually, providing you do not increase your food intake. If you eat less *and* exercise, weight loss will be assured.

Exercising can be as mild as a brisk, daily walk. In fact, studies have shown that women who walked at least thirty minutes a day, under no particular dietary restrictions, lost significant weight in one year. Moreover, obese students at the University of Minnesota who walked ninety minutes a day, five days a week, but did not curtail the amount of food they ate lost an average of fourteen pounds in sixteen weeks!

Regular exercise, then, will virtually guarantee that you will lose weight. Exercise together with a change of eating habits will lead to significant and permanent weight loss and will probably lower your blood pressure as well.

Reducing Sodium Consumption

Most Americans consume much more sodium in the form of sodium chloride, or table salt, than is necessary or, indeed, good for them. In Chapter 2, we presented evidence that an excessive intake of sodium may be a cause of high blood pressure. For that reason alone, most people should try to reduce their sodium consumption.

It is especially important that hypertensive patients cut down on sodium. *Too much sodium can undo the effects of antihypertensive drugs.*

The most commonly prescribed antihypertensive drugs are the diuretics—the "water pills." These drugs act by causing sodium to be excreted in the urine. If you are a heavy salt eater, you could counteract the effects of these drugs. But if you make an effort to restrict your sodium intake, you may be able to get by with lower doses.

The other kinds of antihypertensive drugs, with the exception of propranolol, cause sodium to be retained unless a diuretic is also taken to prevent this retention. If you do not cut back on sodium, the extra sodium in your body can raise your blood pressure and so reduce the effectiveness of these drugs. The extra sodium in your body causes you to need larger doses of the drugs to lower your blood pressure.

In order to cut back on sodium, you must learn which foods are high in sodium. Salty foods contain a great deal of sodium. Salt (sodium chloride, which consists of the chemicals sodium and chlorine) is nearly half sodium. One level teaspoon of salt contains 2,300 milligrams of sodium—more than you should consume in an entire day. Therefore, the first step in reducing your sodium consumption is to stop salting your food at the table and during cooking and to avoid salty foods such as pretzels, potato chips, dill pickles and the like. Almost all processed foods, such as canned goods, contain some added salt.

You may feel that you need to salt your food to bring out its flavor. However, the taste for salt is an acquired one and can be unlearned. In just a few weeks after you stop salting your food, your taste buds will become adjusted. Other spices can be used and a little lemon juice may keep food from tasting flat.

Salt is not the only source of sodium in foods. There is often a great deal of sodium in preservatives, taste enhancers such as sodium glutamate, and the like. It is important to become aware of the sodium content of foods. Most so-called salt substitutes are half-and-half mixtures of sodium and potassium chloride. Read the label carefully before buying any salt substitute, as it still may contain considerable sodium. Ignorance can undo your best efforts to reduce your sodium consumption. For example, James Hunt of the Mayo Clinic found that patients who had cut out salt and who thought their diets were nearly sodium-free almost always consumed at least 2,300 milligrams of sodium daily!

It can be extremely difficult to decide which foods are high in sodium simply by tasting them. Foods with high salt content such as pretzels and potato chips are fairly easy to identify. However, many other foods, including pastries, catsup, packaged breakfast cereals, cheese, and ice cream also may contain a great deal of sodium.

The Center for Science in the Public Interest—a watchdog organization based in Washington, D.C.—has found an interesting example of the surprising sodium content of foods. It obtained a list of the sodium content of products served at McDonald's restaurants. The Center reported that, "With the exception of the soft drinks and orange juice, the item served with the least sodium content is the french fries. Those products with higher sodium content include not only the hamburgers and cheeseburgers but also the 'shakes' and 'apple pies'."

Unfortunately, you cannot always tell which processed foods are high in sodium by reading their labels. Because the Food and Drug Administration does not require sodium content to be listed on the labels of most foods, many manufacturers do not list it. The Center for Science in the Public Interest hopes to change this situation. It recently petitioned the Federal Drug Administration for sodium labeling, commenting, "Considering the large numbers of Americans in dire need of information on the sodium content of foods, it is difficult to justify the mandatory inclusion of thiamine, riboflavin, or other micronutrients in nutrition labeling, while leaving consumers ignorant about sodium."

In order to reduce your sodium consumption you should avoid, as much as possible, processed foods. Even some frozen vegetables have sodium added. It is safest to buy fresh vegetables and fruits, as well as fresh, rather than canned, meats and fish. You should also avoid lunch meats and processed cheeses or cheese spreads, because these foods are high in sodium. To aid you in deciding which foods to eat, refer to Appendix A, which lists the sodium content of some fresh and processed foods.

You can get help in learning to reduce your sodium consumption from your local chapter of the American Heart Association. (Chapters and affiliates are given in Appendix E.) In many communities, the American Heart Association sponsors classes in planning low-sodium meals—classes that are free of charge to patients and their families. In these classes, you can ask questions and discuss your diet problems with a dietician or nutritionist. Your physician or your local chapter of the American Heart Association can tell you how to join. If your local Association does not sponsor a class in sodium-restricted diets, it may begin one if there is sufficient demand.

Reducing sodium consumption may require a change in eating habits, but it need not be a painful change. After a period of adjustment, you can learn to live with quite a bit less sodium. However, the whole purpose of the diuretics is to enable you to lead a normal life. You should restrict your sodium consumption as much as you can, but because of the diuretics you do not have to do without sodium entirely. The more you limit your sodium consumption the less medication you may require; yet there comes a point at which severe sodium restriction may affect the quality of your life. In general, we suggest you stop adding salt to your food and restrict your intake of very salty foods. If you want to go beyond that, well and good. If not, you can be assured that the diuretics will take care of the extra sodium you consume.

Relaxing

Perhaps because the term "hypertension" is often mistakenly identified with nervous tension, many people believe that patients bring high blood pressure on themselves by being tense and nervous. They also believe that hypertension can be prevented or even cured if people would learn to relax.

The idea that relaxation can cure high blood pressure is an appealing one, for it seems that learning to relax should be a pleasant change of life-style. Who among us does not at times feel overly stressed and nervous and who does not at times wish he could simply relax and forget his worries? Many people who learn relaxation techniques such as transcendental meditation and yoga say their lives are greatly enriched by these methods. However, *you cannot expect relaxation to lower your blood pressure permanently.*

As we explained in Chapter 2, it is well established that nervous excitement raises blood pressure and relaxation does the opposite. However, these are only temporary changes and medical investigators have not been able to show that relaxation is an effective treatment for true, persistent high blood pressure. If you want to try relaxation techniques, you should consider them at best a supplement to proved methods of treatment, such as the antihypertensive drugs and weight loss.

But, you may say, even if relaxation doesn't lower blood pressure, couldn't it help prevent a heart attack? Once again, the evidence is inconclusive. Some investigators believe that certain tense, nervous individuals—the "type A" personalities—are more likely than the more relaxed "type B" persons to have heart attacks. Others who have studied this problem disagree on this point. It is, in fact, controversial, and what is more important, *no one has shown that relaxation techniques enable people to change their personalities.*

As an example of the kind of negative results investigators are reporting, we will describe a recent experiment conducted by Henry Blackburn of the University of Minnesota. Blackburn wanted to see whether relaxation can affect blood pressure, cholesterol level, or personality type. He therefore recruited forty-seven men with borderline hypertension. For three months, half of these men practiced relaxation each day, whereas the other half did not. Then the groups switched roles. For the next three months, the group that had originally practiced relaxation stopped doing so and the group that had originally not practiced relaxation did so each day.

Blackburn found that "relaxation had *no* effect on systolic or diastolic blood pressure nor on cholesterol levels of the blood nor on behavior pattern." He concluded, "Relaxation response was *not* found to be an effective nonpharmacologic treatment of mild hypertension, or of hypercholesterolemia [high blood cholesterol], or of Type A behavior pattern."

Exercising

Nowadays, exercise is promoted as the great panacea. It facilitates weight loss, it makes people feel good, and it is even said to cure depression. But one thing exercise will not do is lower the blood pressure. However, regular exercise is still extremely useful to the hypertensive patient because of its effect on weight and because it may help prevent heart disease.

For a number of years, medical investigators were not sure whether exercise lowered blood pressure. Their uncertainty was due to contradictory and confusing reports in the medical literature on the effects of exercise on blood pressure.

One difficulty with these reports is that the studies did not always include a group of people who did not exercise. Typically, the investigators would recruit people with high blood pressure and start them on an exercise program. They would then periodically measure the subjects' blood pressures. Often their blood pressures would be lower a few weeks after exercising was started than they had been at the start of the study. This was interpreted as a demonstration of the success of exercise in lowering blood pressure. But it has been known for a long time that, for most people, blood pressure drops when it is measured repeatedly. This drop occurs because people become accustomed to having their blood pressures measured and so become less anxious during the measurement. Without including people who do not exercise in such studies, it cannot be ruled out that the lowered blood pressure is due to the effect of repeated measurement.

When investigators did include in their studies a group of hypertensive people who did not exercise, they found that exercise did not lower blood pressure. For example, Henry Blackburn and Henry L. Taylor, also of the University of Minnesota, recruited 115 men who were at high risk of developing heart disease. These men smoked cigarettes and had high blood pressure or high concentrations of cholesterol in their blood. The men were divided at random into two groups. One group did not exercise. The other group exercised for one hour a day, three days a week. The blood pressures of both groups decreased slightly over a period of time, but the blood pressures of the men who did not exercise decreased just as much as those of the men who did.

Although it can be definitely concluded that exercise does not lower blood pressure, it is still uncertain whether exercise prevents heart attacks. However, many physicians are convinced by a great deal of circumstantial evidence that it does so.

For more than twenty years, medical investigators have searched for proof that exercise prevents heart disease. The difficulties with their studies are typified by one of the first investigations carried out in 1953 by J. N. Morris of the London School of Hygiene and Public Health. Morris compared the incidence of heart disease among conductors with that among drivers in the London Transport System. The conductors walked up and down the aisles and up to the second deck collecting fares. The drivers remained seated during their work. The results showed that the incidence of heart disease was 30 percent lower among the conductors.

Morris's now-famous study had a serious flaw. The men were not randomly assigned to jobs as conductors or drivers. The leaner men chose or were assigned to be conductors. The heavier men chose or were assigned to be drivers. As Morris himself later pointed out, the average girth in relation to height was greater for drivers than for conductors at the time they entered employment. Thus the leaner conductors may have been healthier to begin with and less prone to develop heart disease than were the more obese drivers.

A flaw like that in Morris's experiment could be avoided if researchers were to recruit a large number of people and *randomly* divide them into two groups. One group would exercise regularly. The other would not. There would be no reason to believe that the exercisers were healthier at the start of the study than those who did not exercise. If the exercisers subsequently had less heart disease, it could be assumed that exercise was responsible for this effect.

This sort of study was recommended in the early 1960s by a committee convened by the Heart Disease Control Program of the Public Health Service. A pilot study was subsequently initiated. The pilot study included a total of 385 men between the ages of forty and fifty-nine who were randomly divided into exercise and nonexercise groups.

Unfortunately, this pilot study failed because about half of the participants dropped out of the exercise group by the end of 6 months. It seemed that the younger and healthier men kept exercising whereas the older and less healthy men dropped out.

Valuable information was nonetheless obtained from this pilot study. The investigators learned that people generally cannot be coerced or persuaded to exercise regularly over long periods of time. In fact, even a desire to exercise may not be enough. Quite a few men dropped out of the exercise group because of injuries.

On the positive side, there is some indirect evidence that exercise might prevent heart disease. It seems that regular exercise might reduce certain risk factors for heart disease. For example, it may lower blood cholesterol concentrations and it may make cells more sensitive to insulin. In diabetes, which is a risk factor for heart disease, cells are relatively insensitive to insulin.

Exercise also strengthens the heart. It enables it to respond more easily and to pump more blood with each contraction. This strengthening of the heart could be important to people whose coronary arteries are partly blocked by atherosclerosis. It makes it less likely that they will feel chest pain upon exertion and so it improves the quality of their lives. Jeffrey Borer, a young cardiologist at the National Heart, Lung, and Blood Institute, exercises regularly in order to keep his heart strong. "Exercise may or may not prevent me from getting heart disease," he says, "but it will at least make me feel more comfortable if I do get it."

Like any other change in life-style, the decision to exercise requires a real commitment. It is not enough to go out and play tennis, for example, on a few weekends when the weather is good. What is needed is some sort of regular exercise several days each week for the rest of your life. This exercise need not be strenuous and could well be simply a moderately long walk. You could walk at lunch time or you could park your car or get off your bus about a mile from your job and walk the rest of the way. In other words, exercise should become a part of your daily life.

Reducing Alcohol Consumption

Most physicians and most hypertensive patients do not consider alcohol intake to be important in hypertension. They may be mistaken. Arthur Klatsby of the Kaiser-Permanente Medical Center in Oakland, California, recently wrote an article in which he explained that people who drink too much alcohol are likely to develop high blood pressure.

The Framingham Study showed that people who consumed 60 or more ounces of alcohol each month were twice as likely to have hypertension as those who consumed less than 30 ounces (900 ml) of alcohol each month. Sixty ounces (1.8 l) of alcohol (200 proof) each month translates into an average daily consumption of 5 ounces (150 ml) of 80 proof spirits, or 16 ounces (480 ml) of table wine, or five 12-ounce (360 ml) bottles of beer. Klatsby enumerates a number of other studies that supported similar conclusions.

What then is a "safe" amount of alcohol to drink? Klatsby suggests that as much as two drinks a day is probably not harmful. *If you consume more than two drinks each day, you should cut back on your alcohol consumption.* A "drink" is a 12-ounce bottle of beer, from 3 to 4 ounces of table wine, or 1 ounce of 80 proof distilled spirits. Most cocktails contain at least 1½ ounces of distilled spirits.

Consuming Caffeine

There is no evidence that caffeine-containing drinks, such as coffee, tea, and colas, contribute to hypertension. A few years ago, it was reported that coffee drinkers are more likely to develop heart disease, but that report has not been confirmed.

Stopping Smoking

Smoking cigarettes does not seem to lead to hypertension and stopping smoking will not lower your blood pressure. There is, however, one very important reason why people with high blood pressure should not smoke. Both smoking and high blood pressure predispose people to develop heart disease. When the two are combined, the risk of heart disease is greatly magnified. For example, the death rate for middle-aged men who have hypertension but no other risk factors for heart disease is twice as high over the next ten years as it is for men with normal blood pressure and no risk factors. If the men also smoke cigarettes, their risk of dying is more than tripled.

Some people are able to stop smoking by themselves, but others find that they need the help of a commercial group such as Smokenders or of a class held by a nonprofit organization such as the American Cancer Society.

In sum, we recommend that you change your eating habits so that you lose weight if you are overweight and that you reduce your sodium consumption. You should engage in moderate exercise at least several times each week, you should drink only in moderation, and you should stop smoking cigarettes if you now smoke them. Although these changes often are not easy to make, they will pay huge dividends in the future and may actually make you feel better now.

APPENDIX A

SODIUM CONTENT OF COMMON FOODS

Approximate Sodium Content of Some Common Foods

Food	Amount	Sodium (milligrams)
Apple	1	2
Bacon (Oscar Meyer), cooked	2 slices	285
Banana	1	1
Beans, baked red kidney (B&M)	1 cup	810
Beans, green, canned (Del Monte)	1 cup	925
Bologna (Oscar Meyer)	2 slices	450
Bread, white (Wonder)	2 slices	297
Bread, whole wheat (Pepperidge Farm)	2 slices	214
Broccoli, frozen (Birds Eye)	1 cup	30
Butter	1 tb	46
Catsup (Heinz)	1 tb	182
Cereal, corn flakes (General Mills)	1 oz	305
Cereal, shreaded wheat (Nabisco)	1 oz	1
Cheese, cheddar (Kraft)	2 oz	380
Cheese, pasteurized processed American (Kraft)	2 oz	890
Cookies, chocolate chip (Pillsbury)	3	130
Cookies, sugar (Pillsbury)	3	210
Frankfurter, beef (Oscar Meyer)	1	425
Ice cream	1 cup	84
Juice, orange	1 cup	2
Juice, tomato (Del Monte)	1 cup	640
Milk, whole	1 cup	122
Mustard (Heinz)	1 tb	213
Pancakes (Hungry Jack Complete)	3 (4-inch)	1,150
Peaches, canned (Del Monte)	1 cup	20
Peanut butter (Jiff)	2 tb	178
Peanuts, unsalted	10	2
Pickle, dill	1 large	1,928
Pizza, frozen (Celeste)	2 oz	328
Potato, baked	1	6
Potato chips (Wonder)	1 oz	220
Pretzel sticks, Mister Salty, Veri-Thin (Nabisco)	1 oz	892
Pudding, instant chocolate (Jell-O)	½ cup	486
Rolls, Danish cinnamin with raisins (Pillsbury)	1 serving	630
Soup, chicken noodle (Campbells)	10 oz prepared	950
Soup, tomato (Campbells)	10 oz prepared	1,050

Food	Amount	Sodium (milligrams)
Soy sauce	1 tb	1,320
Tuna, in oil (Del Monte)	3 oz	430
Turkey, roasted	3 oz	70
Turkey, three-course frozen dinner (Swanson)	17 oz	1,735
Twinkies (Hostess)	1	241

SOURCE: Center for Science in the Public Interest.

NOTE: In general, competing brands contain the same amounts of sodium. Thus, nothing is gained by selecting one brand over another.

APPENDIX B

HOW TO TAKE YOUR OWN BLOOD PRESSURE

Chapter 1 contains a general description of the blood pressure manometer and the principle by which it measures the blood pressure. That section should be read before proceeding further.

There are two main types of instruments, the mercury column and the aneroid. The latter is more compact because the pressure is read by a moving needle on the face of a small circular dial. Never buy an aneroid that has a pin-stop to prevent the needle from falling below zero because one of the checks on the accuracy of the instrument is to see if the needle rests on zero pressure when all of the air is released from the cuff. Although there are very good aneroid manometers, the mercurial type tends to be more dependable, especially in the less-expensive instruments. In general, if you can afford it, the leading American brands, such as Baummanometer or Taylor, are the most reliable and will last the longest with continued use. However, a careful buyer can obtain a good imported instrument at considerably less cost. It is advisable to seek out a large and well-established medical supply store in your area. They generally have the best selection and they also have a reputation to maintain.

The stethoscope, which is used for listening for the sounds over the brachial artery, is also available in several types and at various prices. The Bowles type has a flat, waferlike diaphragm that is pressed over the artery. The bell type stethoscope has a funnel-shaped device for the same purpose. In addition, there are many double-headed or triple-headed stethoscopes that are so designed that cardiologists can listen for murmers over the heart. All these types of instruments are connected to earpieces by means of rubber or plastic tubing. For your purpose, the best purchase is the simplest and least-expensive type of Bowles stethoscope that you can find.

After you have purchased your equipment, you should take it to your physician or his nurse to have it checked. Your blood pressure should be taken several times, first with the physician's professional instrument and then with yours. Allow for a little variation due to changes in blood pressure between readings. If the variation in systolic or diastolic blood pressure is more than 10 mm Hg after several measurements with the two instruments, your manometer is probably defective and should be returned to the dealer.

Providing your equipment tests out satisfactorily, you are ready to learn how to measure blood pressure. If possible, it is far better to have another member of your family be operator of the instrument. You should be seated comfortably with your right arm bared and resting at heart level on a table or desk. The operator should then apply the cuff with the bulb and tubing hanging below the cuff. The cuff should be applied smoothly and snugly but not excessively tightly to the arm so that the lower edge of the cuff is one or two inches above the bend of the elbow. While the cuff is held on the arm with one hand, the loose end should be wrapped around the arm with the other hand and fastened. The type of fastening varies with different instruments, but it is usually a Velcro fastener, which is the easiest to use. Check to see that the cuff overlaps evenly, that it feels comfortable on the arm but is not loose, and that it contains no wrinkles or areas of unevenness.

The operator should now feel with his thumb for the pulsations of your brachial artery. You should have your arm rotated so that the inner side of the elbow and the palm of your hand are facing upward. The operator slides four fingers under the forearm just below the elbow while the thumb remains over the forearm. This allows him to gently but firmly squeeze the forearm between the thumb and fingers because the pulsations are best felt with deep pressure. The pulse is generally felt just below the elbow and in the midline of the long axis of the forearm or just inside (body side) of the midline. The operator should keep moving his thumb about in this area until he feels the strongest pulsation. The stethoscope head should then be placed over this spot and held there by the thumb and fingers of the left hand if the operator is right handed. If he fails to find the pulse, he should repeat the process applying more pressure. In general, the bigger and fatter the arm, the greater is the pressure required to feel the pulse.

Having located the strongest pulsation and having placed the stethoscope firmly and exactly over this spot, the operator should insert the earpieces into his ears, taking care that the curved ends of the earpieces point forward. He is now ready to inflate the rubber bladder inside the cuff. First, he screws the valve of the inflation bulb shut by turning the small metal knob until it can be turned no further. Air can now enter the bladder inside the cuff but cannot leak backward out of the valve. The bladder is then inflated by squeezing the inflation bulb repeatedly. At the same time, the operator watches the mercury column or the needle of the aneroid dial. The operator will note that, after the pressure within the bladder rises above diastolic blood pressure, the mercury or the needle indicator will bounce slightly with each pulsation. At the same time, thumping sounds will be heard in the stethoscope with each pulsation. The operator continues to inflate the cuff until the bouncing motion of the indicator stops and he no longer hears sounds. He proceeds to inflate the bladder until the pressure rises to about 20 or 30 mm Hg above this point.

With his eyes on the manometer scale, the operator opens the valve slightly, allowing the air to leak out slowly. The rate at which the pressure falls should be about 2 or 3 mm Hg per second. If it is faster than this, it is very difficult to determine accurately the point at which the sounds begin. If the rate of deflation is slower than this, the constricting cuff squeezing on the arm will become painful, which in itself will cause the patient's blood pressure to rise. The greatest difficulty that beginners have is to regulate the valve so that the bladder pressure falls gradually but not too slowly. The best way to learn how to do this is to hold the valve control knob between the thumb and forefinger and roll the knob slightly back and forth quickly until the proper rate of decrease is achieved.

As the pressure falls, the operator will begin to hear a thumping sound with each pulsation of the artery. The systolic pressure is the point on the mercury column or the indicator dial at which the pulsations are first heard. As the pressure drops further, the sounds grow louder and then assume a sharp staccato quality; then they suddenly become faint and in a short time disappear. The point at which the sounds disappear is the diastolic blood pressure.

The valve is then opened wide to relieve all pressure on the patient's arm and the systolic and diastolic blood pressures are jotted down. For example, if the sounds began at 152 mm Hg and disappeared at 94 mm Hg, the blood pressure is recorded as 152/94 mm Hg. After a short rest, the procedure can be repeated, as it is more accurate to take the average of several readings.

Although the procedure may sound complicated, it is actually very simple. Almost anyone can learn to take blood pressure. A beginner may be awkward and slow at first, but with a little practice the procedure can be quickly learned.

Some patients prefer to take their own blood pressures or are forced to do so by circumstances. Because it is not easy to relax when occupied with taking the recording, the readings may be higher than they would be if another person were to operate the instrument. Nevertheless, taking one's own blood pressure is an acceptable procedure and supplies useful information.

Cuffs have been prepared especially for the patient who must record his own blood pressure. Unlike the wraparound kind, these cuffs are complete circles that are slipped up the arm. When purchasing this type of cuff, you must be sure that the cuff fits your upper arm snugly but not tightly. Therefore, you should try each one on your arm before you buy any instrument.

Some of these cuffs have the stethoscope head or diaphragm built right into the cuff. If you purchase one of this type, the cuff should be slipped on the arm so that the diaphragm lies under the inside (body side) edge of the biceps muscle in the lower part of the upper arm. If you press deeply in that area with your thumb, you will feel the pulsation of the artery. The earpieces and tubing of the stethoscope are separate. After inserting the earpieces in your ears, screw in the end of the tubing into the connector to the diaphragm. You are now ready to take the blood pressure.

Grasp the bulb and begin to raise the pressure in the cuff. The blood pressure is recorded in exactly the same way as has already been described, except that you are both the operator and the patient. It will take some practice to stay relaxed while you are concentrating on recording the blood pressure. However, most patients seem to have no difficulty in learning how to take satisfactory and representative blood pressures.

Some patients become remarkably adept at taking their own blood pressures—even those who use wraparound cuffs. A patient using a wraparound cuff, with his left arm outstretched on a table, places the end of the cuff on his arm with his right hand. He then lowers his chin onto the cuff to hold it in place while wrapping the length of the cuff around his arm and fastening it in place with his right hand. The Bowles type stethoscope is then slipped under the lower edge of the cuff where the arterial pulse is felt most strongly. The right hand is now free to inflate the rubber bladder. Although this method can be made to work, we do not advise it for the average patient.

Home blood pressure recording is especially useful for patients who become apprehensive in the physician's office. Some normal patients are labeled hypertensive because the apprehension raises their blood pressures far above their usual range. In the more relaxed atmosphere of the home, the recordings reveal consistently normal levels of blood pressure. Obviously, no drug treatment is needed in such cases. Another advantage is for patients who are already under treatment. The frequent home recordings provide a much more accurate index of the effectiveness of treatment than do occasional visits to the physician's office. Furthermore, it is possible to determine whether certain symptoms such as weakness and fatigue are due to excessively low blood pressure caused by the drugs and whether doses of the drugs should be reduced.

In the experience of one of us (Freis), the most knowledgeable patients and the ones in whom the disease is generally best controlled are those who take their blood pressures at home. Nevertheless, there are high-strung patients who become emotionally upset over taking their own blood pressures and there are others who become so obsessed with their readings that they spend a large part of the day recording their blood pressures. For these reasons, some physicians prefer to have their patients abstain from recording their own blood pressures. Thus, a patient should not purchase his own instrument without first obtaining the approval of his personal physician.

APPENDIX C

RELATIVE COSTS OF MEDICATION

The cost of medication is an important consideration in hypertension because you probably will be requiring some form of drug treatment daily year in and year out. Drug costs vary widely depending on the type of drugs taken and whether they are brand-name drugs or generics. In the United States, newly discovered drugs are marketed under patent rights, which means that the company that discovered and tested a drug has a monopoly on it for as long as the patent right lasts—approximately fifteen years. The purpose of this patent law is to give pharmaceutical companies an incentive to develop new and improved drugs through research. And it has paid off very well. All of the antihypertensive drugs that we have today are the result of research done in the laboratories of drug companies. In countries in which no such incentive is provided by law, not a single useful antihypertensive drug has been produced. However, the costs of staffing and maintaining large research laboratories are very great. Furthermore, the food and drug laws in this country are so strict and so much investigation is required, using both animal and human subjects, that bringing a new drug to the marketing stage from the time of its discovery takes from about seven to ten years or more and costs the company from about $20 to $30 million or more.

To pay for its large research and development programs and to make a profit, a company charges a high price for the new drugs on which it has a monopoly under the patent law. When a patent expires, however, other companies can make their own versions of the drug. These copies of the original drug are called generics. They are often made by smaller companies that are not in the business of developing new drugs and, therefore, have no research departments to maintain. Consequently, their costs are much less, they can afford to charge much less, and you pay much less.

RELATIVE COSTS OF MEDICATION

The patents have expired on such drugs as reserpine and hydrochlorothiazide; therefore, they are available as generics. If your physician writes a prescription for reserpine and you request an inexpensive generic brand rather than Serpasil, the brand name for the original Ciba product, you can save considerable money over the years because the difference in cost is great. On the other hand, if the brand name Serpasil is prescribed, you will have no choice but to pay for the Ciba product. Similarly, generic hydrochlorothiazide is much less expensive than the brand names HydroDIURIL or Esidrix.

Although the chemical compound itself is usually the same in both generic and brand-name drugs, there may be other materials added to the brand-name medication that might enhance its absorption, which in some cases may make a considerable difference in its level of activity in the blood. Although this is not true for most generic drugs, if you want to be absolutely on the safe side, you should use the original brand name despite the extra cost.

Obviously, the more recently developed drugs are the most expensive because of the considerations just discussed. Such drugs include alpha methyldopa, clonidine, propranolol, metropolol, and prazosin. They will cost you considerably more than the older drugs. For example, the average cost of treatment with alpha methyldopa is at least ten times as much as the cost of treatment with a generic form of reserpine and at least five times as much as the cost of treatment with the brand name of reserpine, Serpasil.

The retail cost of drugs also varies considerably from one pharmacy to another, depending on how much each pharmacist marks up the price from the wholesale cost. Although generics can vary in quality from one manufacturer to another (and thus from one pharmacy to another), brand-name drugs are identical in quality everywhere. Therefore, you might save considerable money over the years by looking for the best price, especially at the discount pharmacies, before you purchase brand-name drugs. Whether a drug is prescribed by the generic or brand name can be determined by looking it up in Appendix D or by asking your physician.

APPENDIX D

COMMON ANTIHYPERTENSIVE DRUGS

Drug Classification (generic names)	Trade or Brand Name
DIURETICS	
Thiazide and related diuretics	
Chlorothiazide	Diuril
Hydrochlorothiazide	HydroDIURIL, Esidrix, Oretic
Hydroflumethiazide	Saluron
Bendroflumethiazide	Naturetin
Trichlormethiazide	Naqua, Methahydrin
Methyclothiazide	Enduron
Benzthiazide	Exna
Polythiazide	Renese
Cyclothiazide	Anhydrin
Chlorthalidone	Hygroton
Quinethazone	Hydromax
Metolazone	Zaroxolyn
Loop diuretics	
Furosemide	Lasix
Ethacrynic acid	Edecrin
Potassium-sparing diuretics	
Spironolactone	Aldactone
Triamterene	Dyrenium
INHIBITORS OF THE SYMPATHETIC NERVOUS SYSTEM	
Propranolol hydrochloride	Inderal
Metropol	Lopressor
Methyldopa	Aldomet
Clonidine	Catapres
Rauwolfia derivatives	
Reserpine	Serpasil, Sandril
Whole root	Raudixin
Alseroxylon	Rauwiloid
Guanethidine	Ismelin
Prazosin	Minipres

Drug Classification (generic names)	Trade or Brand Name
VASODILATORS	
Hydralazine	Apresoline
COMBINATION DRUGS	
Hydrochlorothiazide + triamterene	Dyazide
Hydrochlorothiazide + reserpine	Hydropres
Hydrochlorothiazide + methyldopa	Alduril
Hydrochlorothiazide + guanethidine	Esimil
Hydrochlorothiazide + hydralazine	Hydralazide, Apresazide
Hydrochlorothiazide + reserpine + hydralazine	Ser-Ap-Es
Chlorthalidone + clonidine	Combipres
Chlorthalidone + reserpine	Regroton

APPENDIX E

AMERICAN HEART ASSOCIATION, INC.

Affiliates and Chapters by State and City

Alabama

Alabama Heart Assn. (Affiliate)
706½ South 29th St.
P.O. Box 31085
Birmingham AL 35222

Alaska

Alaska Heart Assn. (Affiliate)
211 East 4th Ave.
Anchorage AK 99501

Arizona

American Heart Assn.
Arizona Affiliate
1445 East Thomas
Phoenix AZ 85014

Arkansas

Arkansas Heart Assn. (Affiliate)
909 West 2nd St.
P.O. Box 1610
Little Rock AR 72203

California

Kern County Heart Assn. (Chapter)
2628 Eye St.
P.O. Box 2111
Bakersfield CA 93303

San Mateo County Heart Assn. (Chapter)
1848 El Camino Real
Burlingame CA 94010

Ventura County Heart Assn. (Chapter)
1375 Del Norte Rd.
Camarillo CA 93010

American Heart Assn.
Central Valley Chapter
3835 North West Ave.
Fresno CA 93705

Long Beach Heart Assn. (Chapter)
2242 Long Beach Blvd.
Long Beach CA 90806

American Heart Assn.
Greater Los Angeles Affiliate
2405 West 8th St.
Los Angeles CA 90057

Alameda County Heart Assn. (Chapter)
11200 Golf Links Rd.
Oakland CA 94605

American Heart Assn.
Riverside County Chapter
4175 Brockton Ave.
P.O. Box 328
Riverside CA 92506

American Heart Assn.
Golden Empire Chapter
1401 21st St., Suite 306
P.O. Box 160126
Sacramento CA 95816

Central Mission Trails Heart Assn. (Chapter)
600 South Main St.
Salinas CA 93901

San Bernardino County Heart Assn. (Chapter)
960 North D St.
P.O. Box 210
San Bernardino CA 92402

San Diego County Heart Assn. (Chapter)
3640 5th Avenue
San Diego CA 92103

American Heart Assn.
California Affiliate
1370 Mission St.
San Francisco CA 94103

San Francisco Heart Assn. (Chapter)
259 Geary St.
San Francisco CA 94102

Santa Clara County Heart Assn. (Chapter)
1605 The Alameda
San Jose CA 95126

Marin County Heart Assn. (Chapter)
1363 Lincoln Ave.
P.O. Box 15
San Rafael CA 94902

Orange County Heart Assn. (Chapter)
1043 Civic Center Drive West
P.O. Box 1704
Santa Ana CA 92702

American Heart Assn.
Santa Barbara & San Luis Obispo Counties Chapter
223 East De la Guerra St.
P.O. Box 636
Santa Barbara CA 93102

Heart Assn. of the Redwood Empire (Chapter)
4000 Montgomery Dr.
P.O. Box 844
Santa Rosa CA 95405

Central California Heart Assn. (Chapter)
1111 West Robinhood Dr.
Stockton CA 95207

Contra Costa County Heart Assn. (Chapter)
1440 Crokaerts Rd.
P.O. Box 4605
Walnut Creek CA 94596

Colorado

Colorado Heart Assn. (Affiliate)
4521 East Virginia Ave.
Denver CO 80222

Connecticut

Greater Bridgeport Heart Assn. (Chapter)
185 Park Ave.
Bridgeport CT 06604

Connecticut Heart Assn. (Affiliate)
234 Murphy Rd.
Hartford CT 06114

The Heart Assn. of Greater Hartford Inc. (Chapter)
310 Collins St.
Hartford CT 06105

Heart Assn. of Central Conn. Inc. (Chapter)
55 Broad St.
P.O. Box 888
Middletown CT 06457

Heart Assn. of Greater New Haven Inc. (Chapter)
1184 Chapel St.
P.O. Box 1673
New Haven CT 06507

American Heart Assn.
Southwestern Connecticut Chapter
15 Bettswood Rd.
Norwalk CT 06851

Heart Assn. of Eastern Conn. Inc. (Chapter)
88 Main St.
Norwich CT 06360

Heart Assn. of Northwest Conn. Inc. (Chapter)
70 Linden St.
Waterbury CT 06787

Delaware

Delaware Heart Assn. (Affiliate)
Independence Mall, Suite 46
1601 Concord Pike
Wilmington DE 19803

District of Columbia

Washington D.C. Heart Assn. (Affiliate)
D.C. Medical Society Bldg.
2007 Eye St. NW
Washington DC 20006

Florida

Heart Assn. of Broward County Inc. (Chapter)
440 North Andrews Ave.
Fort Lauderdale FL 33301

Northeast Florida Heart Assn. Inc. (Chapter)
1561 San Marco Blvd.
P.O. Box 10022
Jacksonville FL 32207

Heart Assn. of Greater Miami Inc. (Chapter)
5080 Biscayne Blvd.
Miami FL 33137

West Florida Heart Assn. Inc. (Chapter)
105 Santa Rosa Blvd.
Okaloosa Island, Fort Walton Beach FL 32548

Central Florida Heart Assn. Inc. (Chapter)
237 East Marks St.
Orlando FL 32803

Florida Heart Assn. Inc. (Affiliate)
2828 Central Ave.
P.O. Box 10100
St. Petersburg FL 33733

Suncoast Heart Assn. Inc. (Chapter)
3631 5th Ave. North
P.O. Box 12407
St. Petersburg FL 33733

Hillsborough County Heart Assn. (Chapter)
116-A South Howard Ave.
Tampa FL 33606

Canaveral Area Heart Assn. (Chapter)
3435 South Hopkins Ave.
Titusville FL 32780

Heart Assn. of Palm Beach County Inc. (Chapter)
205 Datura St.
West Palm Beach FL 33401

Georgia

Georgia Heart Assn. (Affiliate)
Broadview Plaza, Level C
2581 Piedmont Rd. NE
Atlanta GA 30324

Hawaii

American Heart Assn. of Hawaii Inc. (Affiliate)
245 North Kukui St.
Honolulu HI 96817

Idaho

Idaho Heart Assn. (Affiliate)
2309 Mountain View Dr., Suite 110
Boise ID 83704

Illinois

Chicago Heart Assn. (Affiliate)
22 West Madison St.
Chicago IL 60602

Illinois Heart Assn. (Affiliate)
1181 North Dirksen Parkway
P.O. Box 2666
Springfield IL 62708

Indiana

American Heart Assn.
Northeast Indiana Chapter Inc.
4003 South Wayne Ave.
Ford Wayne IN 46807

American Heart Assn.
Indiana Affiliate Inc.
Missions Bldg., Suite 222
222 South Downey
Indianapolis IN 46219

American Heart Assn.
Marion County Chapter
615 North Alabama St., Room 104
Indianapolis IN 46204

Iowa

Iowa Heart Assn. (Affiliate)
3810 Ingersoll Ave.
Des Moines IA 50312

Kansas

Kansas Heart Assn. (Affiliate)
5229 West 7th St.
Topeka KS 66606

Kentucky

Heart Assn. of Louisville & Jefferson Co. Inc. (Chapter)
207 Speed Bldg.
333 Guthrie St.
Louisville KY 40202

Kentucky Heart Assn. (Affiliate)
207 Speed Bldg.
333 Guthrie St.
Louisville KY 40202

Louisiana

American Heart Assn. of Louisiana Inc. (Affiliate)
3303 Tulane Ave.
P.O. Box 19122
New Orleans LA 70119

Maine

Maine Heart Assn. (Affiliate)
20 Winter St.
Augusta ME 04330

Maryland

American Heart Assn.
Central Maryland Chapter Inc.
415 North Charles St.
Baltimore MD 21202

American Heart Assn.
Maryland Affiliate Inc.
10 South St., Suite 100
Baltimore MD 21201

American Heart Assn.
Montgomery County, Maryland Chapter
7847 Old Georgetown Rd.
Bethesda MD 20014

American Heart Assn.
Western Maryland Chapter Inc.
551 North Centre St.
P.O. Box 1114
Cumberland MD 21502

American Heart Assn.
Frederick/Carroll County, Maryland Chapter
116 East Patrick St.
Frederick MD 21701

Heart Assn. of Southern Maryland (Chapter)
6216 Baltimore Blvd.
Riverdale MD 20840

American Heart Assn. (Chapter)
Maryland Eastern Shore Division
223 East Main St.
Salisbury MD 21801

Massachusetts

American Heart Assn.
Northeast Massachusetts Chapter
79 North Main St.
Andover MA 01810

American Heart Assn.
Massachusetts Affiliate Inc.
85 Devonshire St.
Boston MA 02109

American Heart Assn.
Southeast Massachusetts Chapter
375 Westgate Dr.
Brockton MA 02401

American Heart Assn.
Greater Boston Massachusetts Chapter
112 Cypress St.
Brookline, MA 02146

American Heart Assn.
Cape & Islands Massachusetts Chapter
447 West Main St.
Hyannis MA 02601

American Heart Assn.
Western Massachusetts Chapter
85 Oakland St.
Springfield MA 01108

American Heart Assn.
Central Massachusetts Chapter
9 Exchange St.
Worcester MA 01608

Michigan

Michigan Heart Assn. (Affiliate)
16310 West Twelve Mile Rd.
Box LV 160
Southfield MI 48076

Minnesota

Minnesota Heart Assn. (Affiliate)
4701 West 77th St.
Minneapolis MN 55435

Mississippi
Mississippi Heart Assn. (Affiliate)
4830 East McWillie Circle
P.O. Box 16063
Jackson MS 39206

Missouri
Missouri Heart Assn. (Affiliate)
601 East Broadway
P.O. Box Q
Columbia MO 65201

American Heart Assn.
Kansas City Chapter
616 East 63rd St.
Kansas City MO 64111

St. Louis Heart Assn. (Chapter)
Daudt Memorial Bldg.
4643 Lindell Blvd.
St. Louis MO 63108

Montana
Montana Heart Assn. (Affiliate)
Professional Bldg.
510 1st Ave. North
Great Falls MT 59401

Nebraska
Nebraska Heart Assn. (Affiliate)
3624 Farnam
Omaha NB 68131

Nevada
Nevada Heart Assn. (Affiliate)
455 West 5th St.
Reno NV 89503

New Hampshire
New Hampshire Heart Assn. (Affiliate)
54 South State St.
Concord NH 03301

New Jersey
Camden County Heart Assn. Inc. (Chapter)
7645 Maple Ave.
Pennsauken NJ 08110
726 Cooper St.
Camden NJ 08102

Essex County Heart Assn. (Chapter)
70 East Park St.
East Orange NJ 07017

American Heart Assn.
Union County Chapter
98 West Jersey St.
Elizabeth NJ 07201

American Heart Assn.
Tri-County Chapter
32 East High St.
Glassboro NJ 08028

Bergen County Heart Assn. Inc. (Chapter)
214 Main St.
Hackensack NJ 07601

American Heart Assn.
Middlesex County Chapter
9 South Adelaide Ave.
Highland Park NJ 08904

American Heart Assn.
Monmouth County Chapter
392 Ocean Ave.
Long Branch NJ 07740

American Heart Assn. Morris-Sussex Chapter
9 Pocono Rd.
Denville NJ 07834
55 Maple Ave.
Morristown NJ 07960

American Heart Assn.
Passaic County Chapter
714 Broadway
Paterson NJ 07514

American Heart Assn.
South Jersey Shore Chapter
Shore Mall
1391 Black Horse Pike
Pleasantville NJ 08232

Somerset County Heart Assn. Inc. (Chapter)
11 Maple St.
P.O. Box 852
Somerville NJ 08876

Ocean County Heart Assn. (Chapter)
Oakridge Office Bldg.
215 West Locust St.
Toms River NJ 08753

American Heart Assn.
Mercer County Chapter
824 West State St.
Trenton NJ 08638

American Heart Assn.
New Jersey Affiliate
1525 Morris Ave.
Union NJ 07083

New Mexico

New Mexico Heart Assn. (Affiliate)
142 Truman St. NE, Suite D
Albuquerque NM 87108

New York

American Heart Assn.
Broome County New York Chapter Inc.
8 Riverside Dr.
Binghamton NY 13905

Suffolk Heart Assn. Inc. (Chapter)
127 Atlantic Ave.
Blue Point NY 11715

Heart Assn. of Western New York (Chapter)
Statler Hilton Hotel, Suite 255
Buffalo NY 14202

American Heart Assn.
Finger Lakes Chapter Inc.
191 Parrish St.
P.O. Box 105
Canandaigua NY 14424

Southern Tier Heart Assn. Inc. (Chapter)
530 West Church St.
Elmira NY 14905

Heart Assn. of Southwestern New York Inc. (Chapter)
812 Hotel Jamestown Bldg.
Jamestown NY 14701

American Heart Assn.
Mid-Hudson Chapter Inc.
75 Lucas Ave.
Kingston NY 12401

Heart Assn. of Eastern New York Inc. (Chapter)
257 Osborne Rd.
Loudonville NY 12211

American Heart Assn.
Nassau New York Chapter Inc.
365 Willis Ave.
Mineola NY 11501

Orange-Sullivan Heart Assn. Inc. (Chapter)
469 Broadway
Newburgh NY 12550

American Heart Assn.
New York State Affiliate
3 West 29th St.
New York NY 10001

New York Heart Assn. (Affiliate)
2 East 64th St.
New York NY 10021

American Heart Assn.
Dutchess County Chapter Inc.
31 Haight Ave.
Poughkeepsie NY 12603

Westchester Heart Assn. Inc. (Chapter)
Pforzheimer Memorial Bldg.
Purchase St., Rt. 120
Purchase NY 10577

Genesee Valley Heart Assn. (Chapter)
217-A Alexander St.
Rochester NY 14607

American Heart Assn.
Upstate New York Chapter Inc.
1212 James St.
Syracuse NY 13203

Central New York Heart Assn. Inc. (Chapter)
1024 Park Ave.
Utica NY 13502

American Heart Assn.
Northern New York Chapter
1402 Washington St.
Watertown NY 13601

North Carolina

North Carolina Heart Assn. (Affiliate)
1 Heart Circle
P.O. Box 2408
Chapel Hill NC 27514

Heart Assn. of Charlotte & Mecklenburg Co. (Chapter)
1351 East Morehead St.
Charlotte NC 28204

Gaston County Heart Assn. (Chapter)
408 South St.
P.O. Box 877
Gastonia NC 28052

Greensboro Heart Assn. (Chapter)
1600 East Wendover Ave.
P.O. Box 20804
Greensboro NC 27420

Forsyth County Heart Assn. (Chapter)
2046 Queen St.
Winston-Salem NC 27103

North Dakota

American Heart Assn.
Dakota Affiliate Inc.
1005 12th Ave. SE
P.O. Box 1287
Jamestown ND 58401

Ohio

American Heart Assn.
Akron District Chapter Inc.
326 Locust St.
Akron OH 44302

American Heart Assn.
East Central Ohio Chapter Inc.
1341 Cleveland Ave. NW
Canton OH 44703

American Heart Assn.
Southwestern Ohio Chapter Inc.
2831 Vernon Pl.
Cincinnati OH 45219

American Heart Assn.
Northeast Ohio Affiliate
1689 East 115th St.
Cleveland OH 44106

American Heart Assn.
Central Ohio Heart Chapter Inc.
535 East Broad St.
Columbus OH 43215

American Heart Assn.
Ohio Affiliate Inc.
10 East Town St., Room 506
Columbus OH 43215

American Heart Assn.
Miami Valley Heart Chapter Inc.
124 North Jefferson St.
Dayton OH 45402

American Heart Assn.
Northwestern Ohio Chapter Inc.
215 Community Services Bldg.
1 Stranahan Sq.
Toledo OH 43604

American Heart Assn.
Eastern Ohio Chapter Inc.
4822 Market St.
Youngstown OH 44512

Oklahoma

American Heart Assn.
Oklahoma Affiliate
800 Northeast 15th St.
P.O. Box 11376
Oklahoma City OK 73111

American Heart Assn.
Tulsa Chapter
4515 South Yale, Suite 200
Tulsa OK 74135

Oregon

Oregon Heart Assn. (Affiliate)
1500 Southwest 12th Ave.
Portland OR 97201

Pennsylvania

American Heart Assn.
Allegheny Mountain Pennsylvania Chapter
Clearfield Hospital, Nurses Home
P.O. Box 92
Clearfield PA 16830

American Heart Assn.
Southwestern Pennsylvania Chapter
223 North Maple Ave.
Greensburg PA 15601

American Heart Assn.
Pennsylvania Affiliate
2743 North Front St.
P.O. Box 2435
Harrisburg PA 17110

American Heart Assn.
South Central Pennsylvania Chapter
2915 Wayne St.
Harrisburg PA 17111

American Heart Assn.
Pennsylvania Highlands Chapter
408 Lincoln St.
Johnstown PA 15901

American Heart Assn.
Lancaster Pennsylvania Chapter
246 West Orange St.
Lancaster PA 17603

American Heart Assn.
Northwestern Pennsylvania Chapter
902 Diamond Park
P.O. Box 126
Meadville PA 16335

American Heart Assn.
Midwestern Pennsylvania Chapter
109 East North St.
New Castle PA 16101

American Heart Assn.
Southeastern Pennsylvania Chapter
318 South 19th St.
Philadelphia PA 19103

Western Pennsylvania Chapter
4 Smithfield St.
709 House Bldg.
Pittsburgh PA 15222

American Heart Assn.
Keystone Pennsylvania Chapter
730 Pittston Ave.
Scranton PA 18505

American Heart Assn.
Central Pennsylvania Chapter
409 South Allen St.
State College PA 16801

American Heart Assn.
Northeastern Pennsylvania Chapter
Kirby Health Center
71 North Franklin St.
Wilkes-Barre PA 18701

American Heart Assn.
Northcentral Pennsylvania Chapter
1967-69 West 4th St.
Williamsport PA 17701

American Heart Assn.
York-Adams Pennsylvania Chapter
105 South George St.
P.O. Box 494
York PA 17405

Puerto Rico

Puerto Rico Heart Assn. (Affiliate)
Box 8215
Fernandez Juncos Station
Santurce PR 00910

Rhode Island

Rhode Island Heart Assn. (Affiliate)
40 Broad St.
Pawtucket RI 02860

South Carolina

South Carolina Heart Assn. (Affiliate)
2864 Devine St.
P.O. Box 5937
Columbia SC 29205

Tennessee

Chattanooga Area Heart Assn. (Chapter)
519 East 4th St.
Chattanooga TN 37403

West Tennessee Heart Assn. (Chapter)
1023 Campbell St.
P.O. Box 1086
Jackson TN 38301

East Tennessee Heart Assn. (Chapter)
1206 Pierce Parkway
P.O. Box 709
Knoxville TN 37901

Memphis Heart Assn. (Chapter)
28 North Claybrook St.
P.O. Box 4706
Memphis TN 38104

Middle Tennessee Heart Assn. (Chapter)
209 23rd Ave. North
Nashville TN 37203

Tennessee Heart Assn. (Affiliate)
1720 West End Bldg., Suite 308
Nashville TN 37203

Texas

American Heart Assn.
Texas Affiliate Inc.
860 North Highway 183
P.O. Box 15186
Austin TX 78761

Utah

Utah Heart Assn. (Affiliate)
250 East 1st South
Salt Lake City UT 84111

Vermont

Vermont Heart Assn. (Affiliate)
56 Church St.
Rutland VT 05701

Virginia

American Heart Assn.
Northern Virginia Chapter Inc.
609 North Edgewood St.
Arlington VA 22201

American Heart Assn.
Piedmont Chapter Inc.
128 Linden Ave.
Lynchburg VA 24503

American Heart Assn.
Virginia Peninsula Chapter Inc.
627 79th St.
P.O. Box 5009
Newport News VA 23605

American Heart Assn.
Tidewater Chapter Inc.
891 Norfolk Sq.
Norfolk VA 23502

American Heart Assn.
Richmond Area Chapter Inc.
3206 Cutshaw Ave.
Richmond VA 23230

American Heart Assn.
Virginia Affiliate Inc.
316 East Clay St.
Richmond VA 23219

Washington

Washington State Heart Assn. (Affiliate)
333 1st Ave West
Seattle WA 98119

Washington State Heart Assn.
Northeastern Chapter
321 Hutton Bldg.
Spokane WA 99204

West Virginia

American Heart Assn.
West Virginia Affiliate
211 35th St. SE
Charleston WV 25304

Wisconsin
Wisconsin Heart Assn. (Affiliate)
795 North Van Buren St.
Milwaukee WI 53202

Wyoming
Wyoming Heart Assn. (Affiliate)
217 West 18th St.
Cheyenne WY 82001

INDEX